Bone SPECT/CT of Ankle and Foot

Guillaume Chuto · Emmanuel Richelme
Christophe Cermolacce · Michel Nicaud
Bruno Puech

Bone SPECT/CT of Ankle and Foot

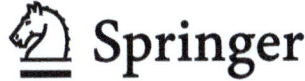 Springer

Guillaume Chuto
Nuclear Physician
Résidence du Parc Clinic
Marseille
France

Michel Nicaud
Nuclear Physician
Résidence du Parc Clinic
Marseille
France

Emmanuel Richelme
Orthopedic Foot and Ankle Surgeon
Juge Clinic
Marseille
France

Bruno Puech
Nuclear Physician
Résidence du Parc Clinic
Marseille
France

Christophe Cermolacce
Orthopedic Foot and Ankle Surgeon
Juge Clinic
Marseille
France

Originally published in French: Tomoscintigraphie osseuse de la cheville et du pied by Guillaume
Chuto et al. © Sauramps Medical 2016. All Rights Reserved.
ISBN 978-3-319-90810-6   ISBN 978-3-319-90811-3   (eBook)
https://doi.org/10.1007/978-3-319-90811-3

Library of Congress Control Number: 2018955312

This Springer imprint is published by the registered company Springer Nature Switzerland AG
The registered company address is: Gewerbestrasse 11, 6330 Cham, Switzerland

Preface

For a long time, foot and ankle imaging was limited to the use of standard x-rays, which remain an indispensable technique today. At the end of the 1980s, computed tomography (CT), magnetic resonance imagery (MRI), and ultrasonography (US) allowed for volume imaging which revolutionized the practice of radiology. Radiologists had to learn a new radiological semiology and face an influx of anatomical and pathological information that had not been visualized previously.

This type of revolution is occurring for the nuclear physicians.

Bone scans carried out by traditional gamma cameras were little used for foot imaging due to their lack of specificity and low anatomical resolution. They were primarily used to diagnose algodystrophy, stress fractures, and acute osteomyelitis in children and to assess foot pain when x-rays were normal. A normal bone scan had a rather good negative predictive value to eliminate an osteoarticular etiology. But in the event of increased tracer uptake, it was often impossible to say if the uptake was on a bone or an articulation, or if ankle uptake revealed a talar or a malleolar problem. Single-photon emission computed tomography (SPECT), allowing the capture of 3D images with detection heads that rotate 360°, was technically feasible but unexploitable due to the small structures of the foot and was thus not used.

At the end of the 2000s, the arrival of hybrid scanners with the ability to acquire SPECT and multislice CT data simultaneously opened a wide range of prospects for the nuclear physicians [1]. Combining SPECT and CT considerably increases bone scan image quality (attenuation correction), anatomic localization, and diagnostic accuracy (improved sensitivity and specificity and a reduction in the number of undetermined tests) [2].

Since 2011, the term "bone SPECT" includes the CT study, and these hybrid scanners allow a three-dimensional analysis particularly helpful for foot evaluation, the foot being a complex structure made up of 26 bones.

At the end of 2012 in France, approximately 150 of the 500 gamma cameras installed were hybrid scanners [3], and their proportion continues to increase, demonstrating the clinical impact of this technological advance.

Like their fellow radiologists at the beginning of the 1990s, nuclear physicians are discovering pathologies previously unknown to them and increased tracer uptake that they couldn't previously see. They must in turn learn a new semiology. This is the objective of this book, which was written by nuclear physicians and orthopedic surgeons specialized in the foot and ankle.

This book has two parts:

- The first part is devoted to pathology. The most frequent ankle and foot pathologies that can be seen with a bone scan are described briefly, with a focus on bone scan data. Sidebars highlight information useful to orthopedic surgeons. Bone scan studies of clinical interest are presented. Certain frequent or useful-to-know pathologies that are not diagnosed by bone scan will be also described (such as Morton's neuroma).
- The second part is devoted to anatomy, covering the bones, joints, and relevant anatomic structures needed to interpret a bone scan of the ankle or foot. They are presented with captioned drawings.

The anatomical nomenclature used is in "Nomina Anatomica," recognized by all the countries.

This book deals with single-photon emission computed tomoscintigraphy (SPECT) with Technetium 99m (^{99m}Tc-HDP), but the data presented can also be used with positron emission tomography (PET) with sodium fluoride-18 (^{18}FNA).

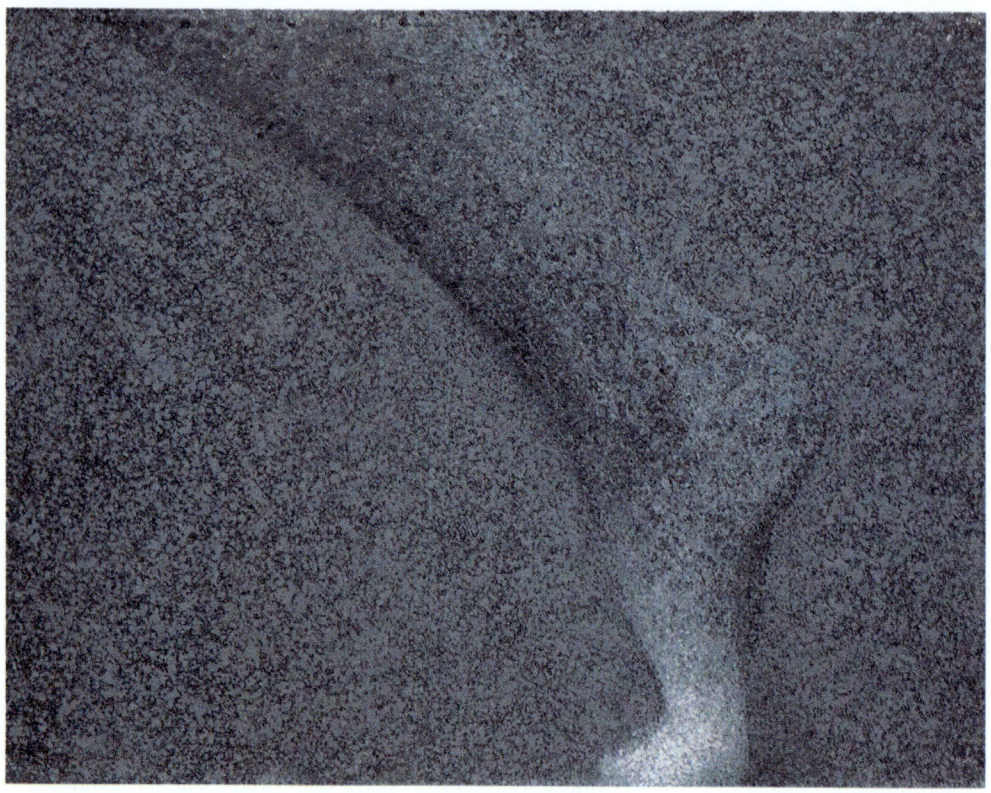

"Taking off" by Jonathan Lane, acrylic resin on paper, 85 × 110 cm, 2015

Marseille, France

Guillaume Chuto
Emmanuel Richelme
Christophe Cermolacce
Michel Nicaud
Bruno Puech

Acknowledgements

The authors would like to thank the following physicians for their precious help:

Cecile Colavolpe
Nuclear Physician
CHU Timone, Marseille

Laurent Tessonnier
Nuclear Physician
CHIC Sainte Musse, Toulon

Marie-Christine Maximin
Orthopedic Pediatric Surgeon
Résidence du Parc Clinic, Marseille

Eric Dobbels
Rheumatologist
Borromées Medical Center, Marseille

Hélène Bonnaure
Diabetes and Endocrinology Specialist
CH Narbonne, Narbonne

Thierry Mirabel
Radiologist
Résidence du Parc Clinic, Marseille

Jean-Charles Grillo
Adult Orthopedic Surgeon
CHIC Sainte Musse, Toulon

Assi Assi
Infectiologist
CHIC Sainte Musse, Toulon

Nicolas Macagno
Anatomopathologist
CHU Timone, Marseille

Antoine Micheau
Radiologist
IMAIOS SAS, Montpellier

Denis Hoa
Radiologist
IMAIOS SAS, Montpellier

The authors would like to thank the staff of the Nuclear Medicine Department at the Résidence du Parc Clinic and the Orthopedic staff at the Juge Clinic for their help with this book.

We would also like to thank Dr. **Isabelle Nicol**, a dermatologist in Marseilles, and Dr. **France Guarrigues**, a general practitioner in Marseilles, for reading the final draft.

Anatomical illustrations are taken from the E-Anatomy Atlas (Copyright ©2008–2015 IMAIOS SAS—all rights of translation, adaptation, and reproduction reserved for all countries.)

The e-Anatomy Atlas is available online on www.imaios.com

Contents

Abbreviations

a.	Artery
Ab	Antibody
ACPA	Anti-citrullinated peptide antibody
ACR	American College of Rheumatology
ant.	Anterior
ATB	Antibiotic
ATCD	Antecedent
ATFL	Anterior talofibular ligament
ATT	Action to be taken
BC	Blood culture
BK	Back
BMB	Bone marrow biopsy
BMI	Body mass index
BMP	Bone morphogenetic protein
BS	Bone scan
C°	Centigrade
CBT	Cognitive behavioral therapy
CIC	Change in conditions
cf	Confer
CFL	Calcaneofibular ligament
cm	Centimeter
CNS	Central nervous system
CRP	C-reactive protein
CRPS 1	Complex regional pain syndrome type 1 (previously referred to as algodystrophy)
CT	Computed tomography
$CTDI_{vol}$	Volume computed tomography dose index
D	Day
DHM	Dietetic and hygiene measures
diabetic NOA	diabetic neuropathic osteoarthropathy
DIP	Distal interphalangeal joint
DIS	Disease
dg	Diagnosis
DLP	Dose-length product
DMARDs	Disease-modifying anti-rheumatic drugs
ESR	Erythrocyte sedimentation rate
EULAR	European League Against Rheumatism
F	Front
fat sat	Fat saturation
FDG	^{18}F-Fluorodeoxyglucose
FHL	Flexor hallucis longus
FNA	^{18}F-sodium fluoride

FX	Fracture
g	Gram
Gd	Gadolinium
HU	Hounsfield Units
ICA	Iodinated contrast agents
inf.	Inferior
IPJ	Interphalangeal joint
IV	Intravenous
lat.	Lateral
lig.	Ligament
LN	Lymph node
M1	First metatarsal
MBq	Megabecquerel
MCP	Metacarpophalangeal articulation
med	Medial
M/F	Male/female ratio
MIP	Maximum Intensity Projection
MRI	Magnetic resonance imaging
MTP	Metatarsophalangeal joint
MUS	Muscle
n.	Nerve
NB	Nota bene
NOA	Nervous osteoarthropathy
NR	Not relevant
NSAIDs	Nonsteroidal anti-inflammatory drugs
NTR	Nothing to report
OLT	Osteochondral lesion of the talus
op.	Operational
P1	1st phalanx
PAD	Peripheral arterial disease
PCR	Polymerase chain reaction
PET	Positron emission tomography
PIP	Proximal interphalangeal joint
PN	Polynuclear neutrophil
PNS	Peripheral nervous system
PO	Per os
post.	Posterior
PsA	Psoriatic arthritis
pso	Psoriatic
RA	Rheumatoid arthritis
RF	Risk factor
Se	Sensitivity
SFX	Stress fracture
Sp	Specificity
sup.	Superior
SUV	Standardized Uptake Value
Sv	sievert
TAP	Total ankle prosthesis
THA	Total hip arthroplasty
TNF	Tumor necrosis factor
TNM	T = primary tumor, N = regional lymph nodes, M = distant metastasis
TS	Tendinous sheath
Tx	Treatment

UC	Ulcerous colitis
V	Vein
WB	Whole body
WBC	White blood cells
WBC count	White blood cells count

Abbreviations in Images

AV *(for "avant")*	Front
AR *(for "arrière")*	Back
D *(for "droite")*	Right
G *(for "gauche")*	Left

Part I

Pathology

Orthopedics

Lateral Ankle Sprain

Predisposition:
- Sports or daily life accident

Past medical history:
- +/− sprains, ankle instability

Frequency [4, 5]:
- The most frequent injury encountered in traumatology
- 6000/D in France

Mechanism:
- The ankle being forced into too much inversion causes injury to the lateral collateral ligament, predominantly impacting the anterior talofibular ligament (++++, **ATFL**), followed by the calcaneofibular ligament (CFL) and finally the superior fibular retinaculum (Fig. 1).

Types: NR
Interview:
- Inversion twist of the ankle
- Usually three phases of pain: intense pain, sedation, and painful recovery

Clinical examination:
- Lateral malleolus hematoma.
- Walking: possible/impossible.
- Palpation: look for signs of fracture (Ottawa ankle rules).
- **Initial clinical examination can be difficult:**
  - Examination in 5 days is more precise for the diagnosis of lateral ankle sprain, ↗ SE and Sp ≈ 85 and 95%, respectively [6].
  - Initial assessment incorrect in 30% of sprains seen in emergency care [4].

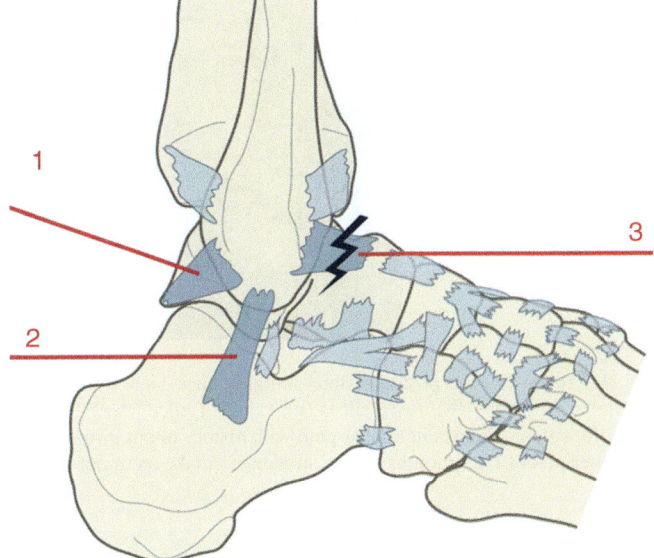

Fig. 1 Lateral ankle sprain. Predominantly impacting the anterior talofibular ligament (black zigzag line). (1) Posterior talofibular ligament (2) Calcaneofibular ligament (3) Anterior talofibular ligament

Paraclinical examination:
- If benign sprain: clinical examination is sufficient.
- If moderate or severe sprain: ultrasound.
- If positive Ottawa ankle rules: X-ray to look for fracture.

Differential:
- There are a number of differential diagnoses and/or related injuries:
  - Malleolus fracture and malleolus avulsion fracture
  - Fracture of the posterior tibial margin (Fig. 2)
  - Fracture of the talus:
    Superolateral fracture of the trochlea of talus
    Fracture of the lateral process
    Fracture of the neck

© Springer International Publishing AG, part of Springer Nature 2018
G. Chuto et al., *Bone SPECT/CT of Ankle and Foot*, https://doi.org/10.1007/978-3-319-90811-3_1

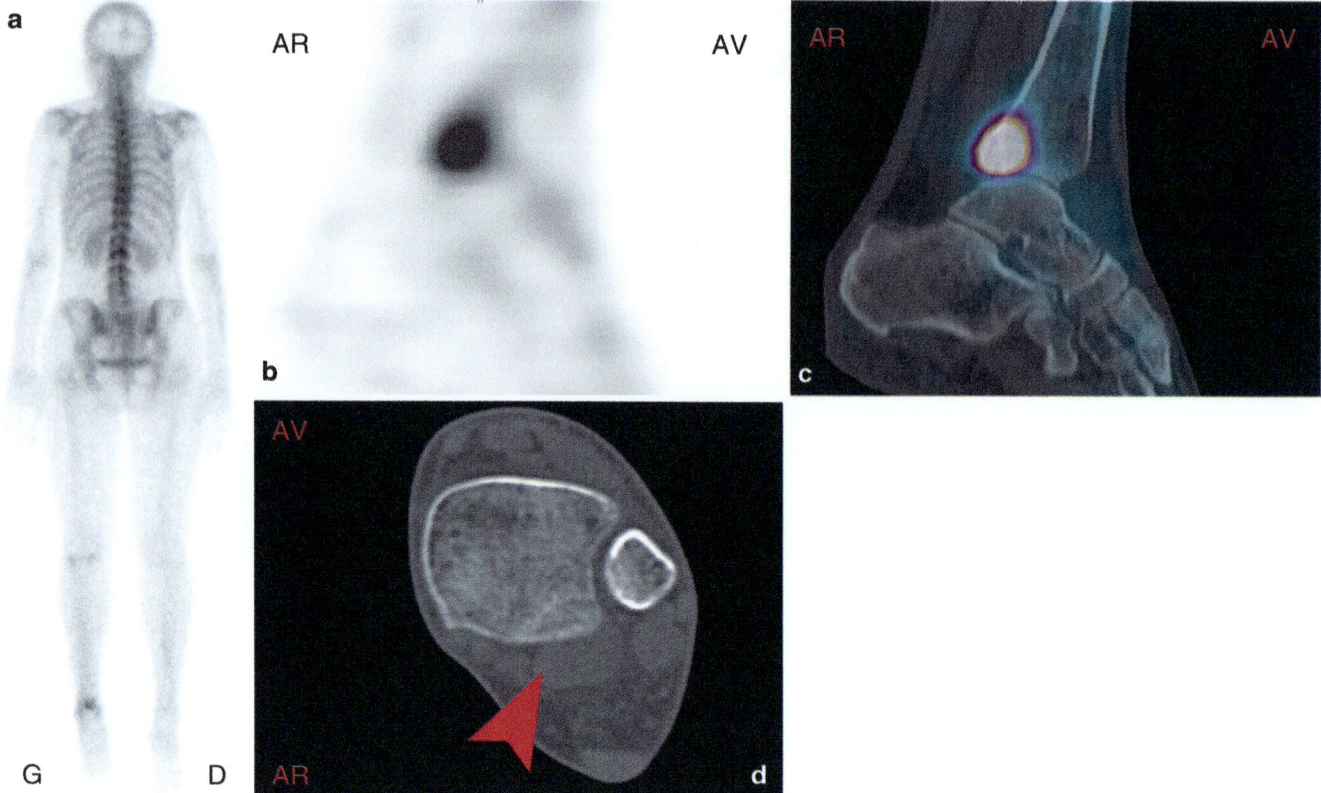

Fig. 2 Fracture of the posterior tibial margin. Back view of WB (**a**), sagittal scintigraphy (**b**), fused slices (**c**), axial CT slice (**d**). Fifty-six-year-old woman, persistent lumbar pain with history of compression of the upper part of L2 5 months earlier: moderate uptake on upper part of L2, isolated and mild (SPECT images not shown). Unexpected uptake in left ankle, still painful following a sprain 2 months prior: non-displaced fracture not seen previously (arrowhead)

– Fifth metatarsal base fracture (fibularis brevis tendon attachment)
– Navicular fracture
– Injury to the ligaments of the transverse tarsal joint
– Injury/dislocation of fibularis tendons
– Injury to anterior tibiofibular ligament +/− interosseous membrane of the leg

Classification: There are different classifications.
• Benign sprain: ecchymotic infiltration of the ligament
• Moderate sprain: partial rupture +/− periosteal stripping
• Severe sprain: complete rupture +/− bone avulsion

Evolution:
• Chronic pain due to:
  – Fibrosis leading to impingement (cf. impingement pages)
  – Lack of ligament healing
  – Diagnostic error/unseen related injury
• Instability: poorly healed severe sprain (Fig. 3)

Treatment [5, 6]:
• Initial consultation and **systematic second assessment between D3 and D5**
• Early Tx, **always followed by functional rehabilitation**
• In cases of functional Tx:
  – No immobilization
  – Rapid return to activity
• Benign sprain:
  – **Functional Tx**, RICE protocol
    Rest
    Ice
    +/− Compression: splint (Aircast type) for a few days
    Elevation
• Moderate sprain:
  – Functional Tx: RICE protocol
    Rest + crutches
    Ice
    +/− Compression: splint (Aircast type) for a few weeks
    Elevation
• Severe sprain:
  – Orthopedic Tx: strict immobilization for 6 weeks
  – Or surgery

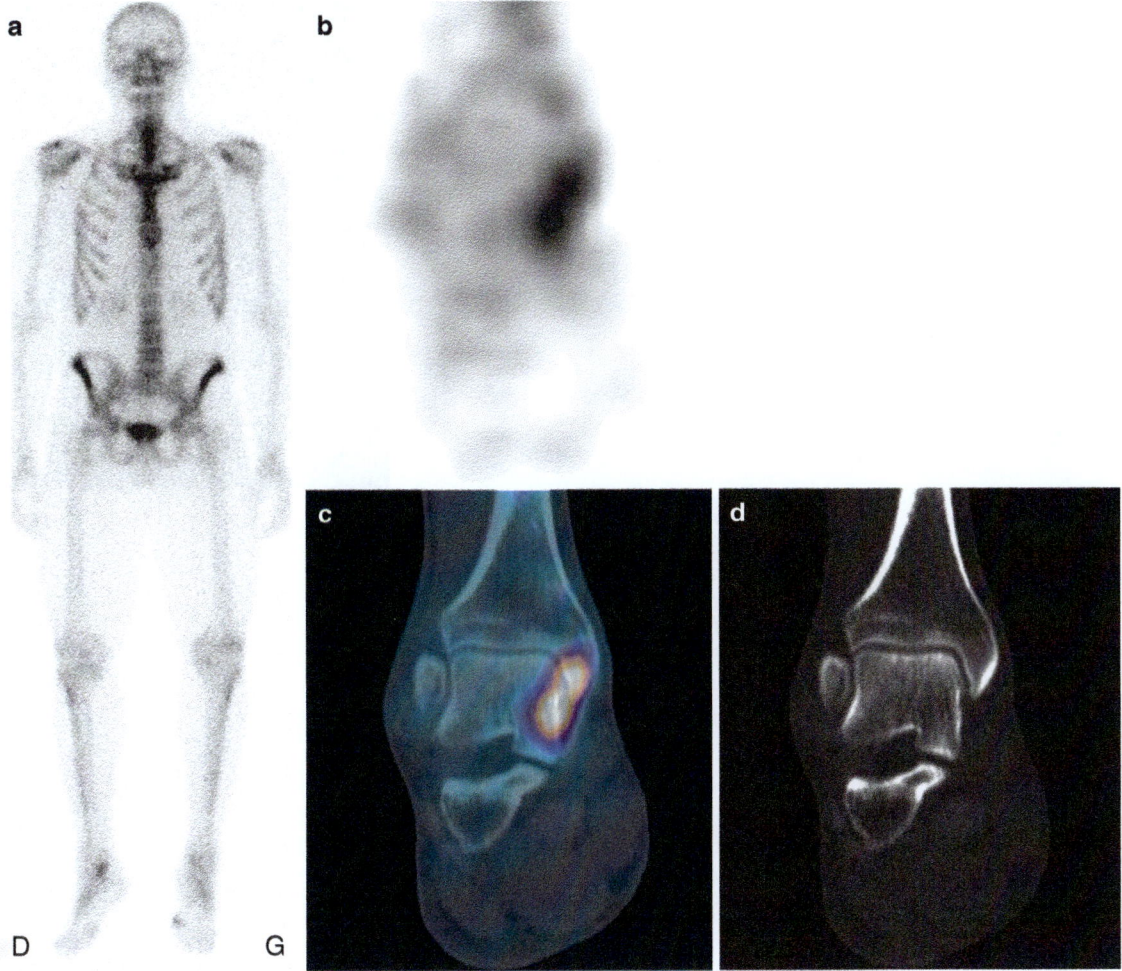

Fig. 3 (**a–d**) Chronic instability of the right ankle with persistent pain following varus sprain 4 months prior. Front view of WB (**a**), frontal SPECT (**b**), fused (**c**), and CT (**d**) slices. Moderate uptake of a contusion between the medial malleolus and the talus occurred during the injury

Discussion:

- A bone scan is not useful during the acute phase of a lateral ankle sprain. It can, however, be useful in the case of early residual pain (undiagnosed avulsion fracture, bone contusion) or chronic pain (OLT) (Figs. 4 and 5).

Box 1
Ottawa ankle rules, X-rays justified if [4, 7, 8]:

- >55 years old
- And/or inability to bear weight for four steps both immediately and in the emergency department
- And/or bone tenderness:
  - On the tip of the lateral malleolus or along the distal 6 cm of the posterior edge of the fibula
  - On the tip of the medial malleolus or along the distal 6 cm of the posterior edge of the tibia
  - At the base of the fifth metatarsal
  - At the navicular

Box 2
The goal of the initial care for a lateral ankle sprain is:

- Assess the severity.
- Look for related injuries.
- Eliminate a differential diagnosis.

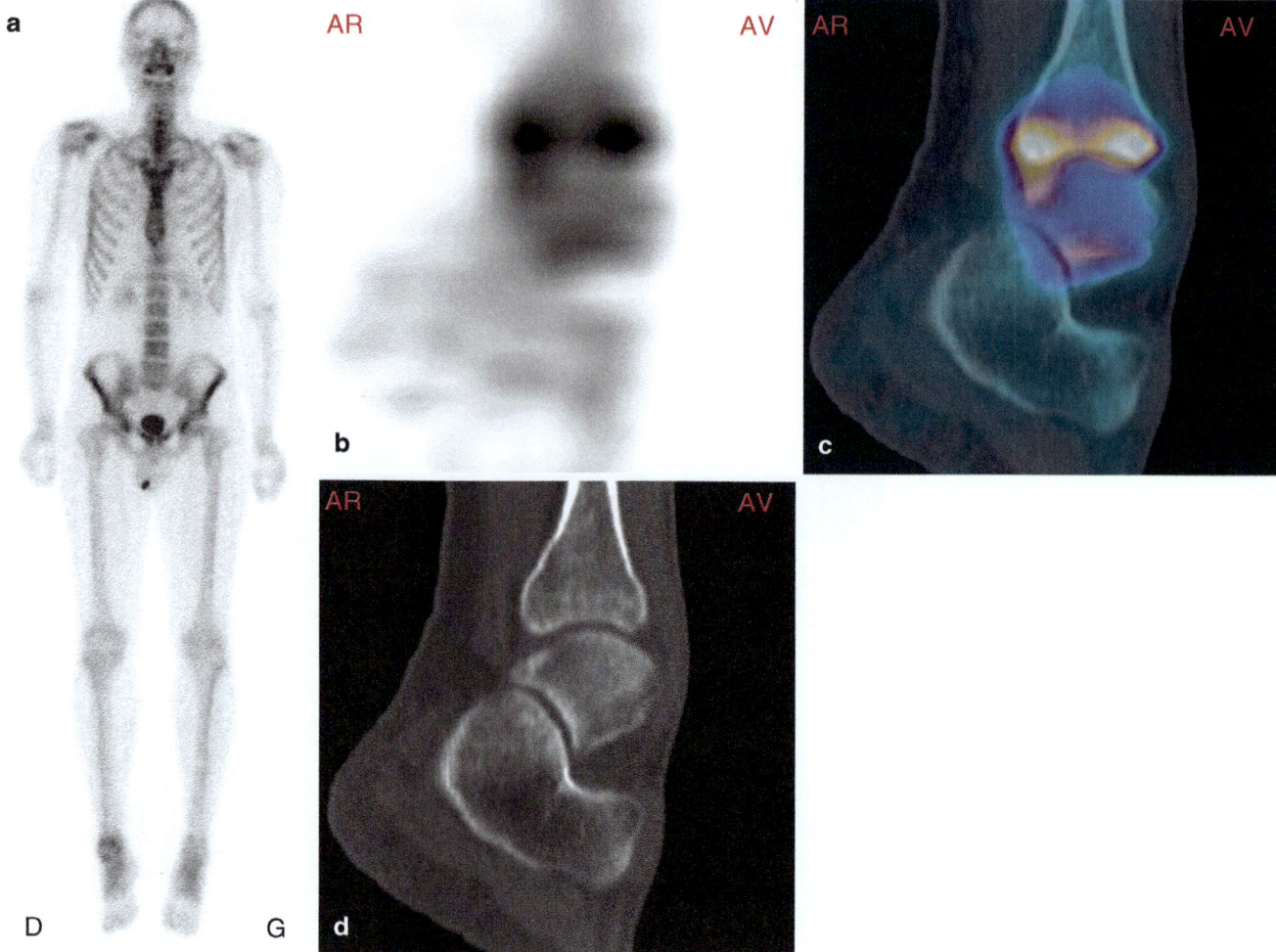

Fig. 4 (**a–d**) Contusion of the lateral tibial margin. Front view of WB (**a**), sagittal SPECT (**b**), fused (**d**), and CT (**d**) slices. Right ankle varus injury 6 months prior, with moderate sprain of the ATFL, treated, persistent pain. Discovery of a contusion that had not been seen previously. Note moderate contusion uptake on the WB image, indicating it is not so recent (6 months), and the lack of anomalies on the CT, which eliminates fractures

Fig. 5 (**a–c**) Bimalleolar contusion. Front view of WB (**a**) and blood pool phase (**b**), fused frontal slice (**c**). Three-month-old right foot sprain, MRI done 2 months prior: ATFL rupture and medial and lateral perimalleolar edema. Persistent pain: note the uptake at each malleolar tip and on the opposite talus. There is no OLT or any ankle arthropathy. The activity on the blood pool phase of the left limb, particularly in the medial part of the ankle, seems to indicate asymptomatic overuse of this limb

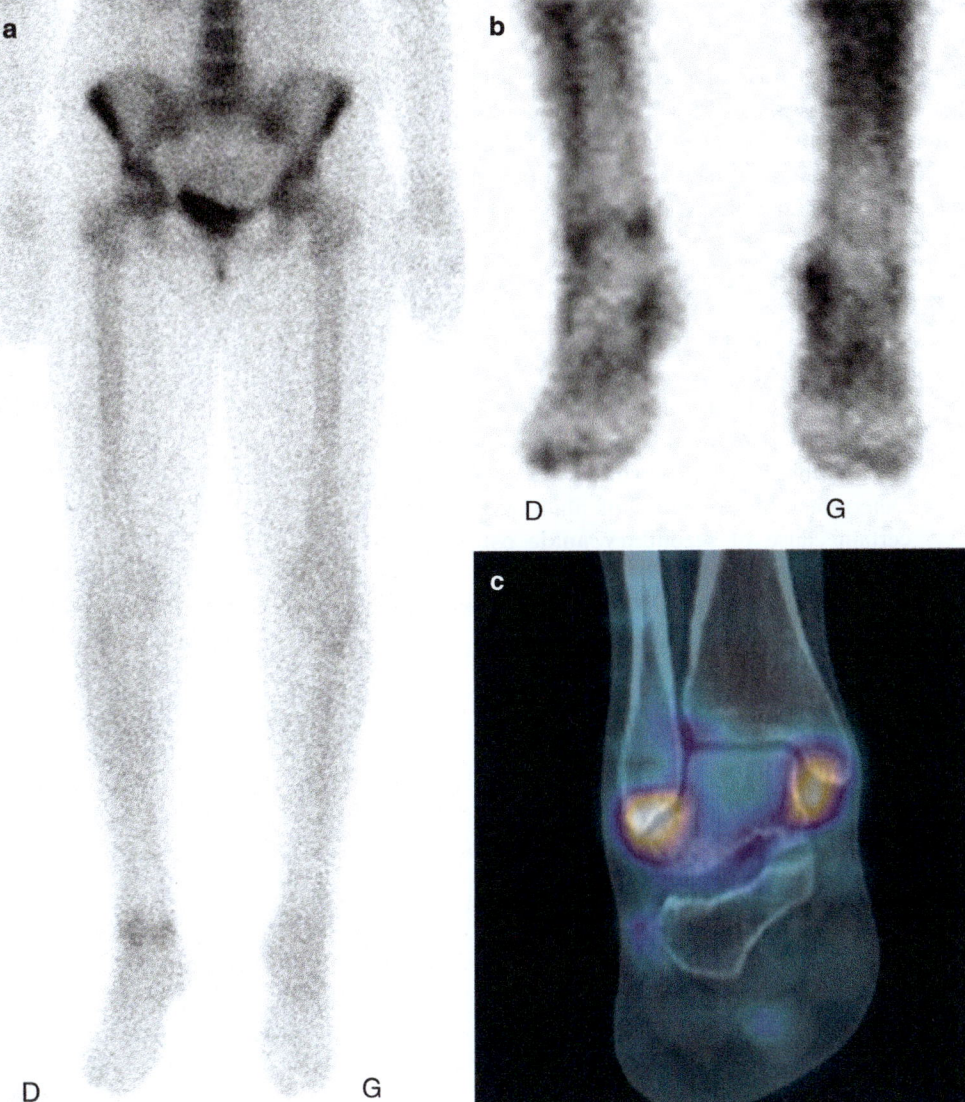

Fractures

The objective of this chapter is not to describe all types of fractures, but to insist on those that are harder to see with standard radiography but can be seen with bone scans (BS) carried out to assess persistent pain after a sprain and to present the fractures whose aftereffects are frequently seen on BS.

Bimalleolar fracture [9, 10]:
- Frequent.
- Valgus (+++) or varus sprain.
- Alnot and Duparc classification (Fig. 6):
  - Based on the injury mechanism and the **base of the fibular line compared to the distal tibiofibular ligaments** (tibiofibular syndesmosis)
  - Determines the existence of tibiofibular **diastasis**, a certain cause of **secondary ankle osteoarthritis** if neglected
- Bimalleolar fractures in which the fibular line is above the syndesmosis lead to tibiofibular diastasis:
  Supraligamentary bimalleolar Fx
  Maisonneuve Fx
  Certain equivalents of bimalleolar Fx

- Look for related injury of the distal tibial margin:
  - Anterior margin
  - Posterior margin (++):
    Frequent, also called a trimalleolar fracture.
    Three types (Fig. 7) [9]: seriousness and treatment depend on the degree to which the articular surface is impacted.
    Type a (extra-articular) and type b (most frequent) do not require specific Tx apart from surgery for the bimalleolar fracture.
- Tx: surgical (+++) (Fig. 8).

Fracture of the distal tibial epiphysis (tibial pilon fracture) [10, 11]:
Fall from a high place
- Articular fracture: high risk of **secondary ankle osteoarthritis**
- Five types of fractures:
  - Posterior margin: can be seen with BS
  - Anterior margin
  - Complex (++)
  - Supra-malleolar with articular propagation
  - Sagittal

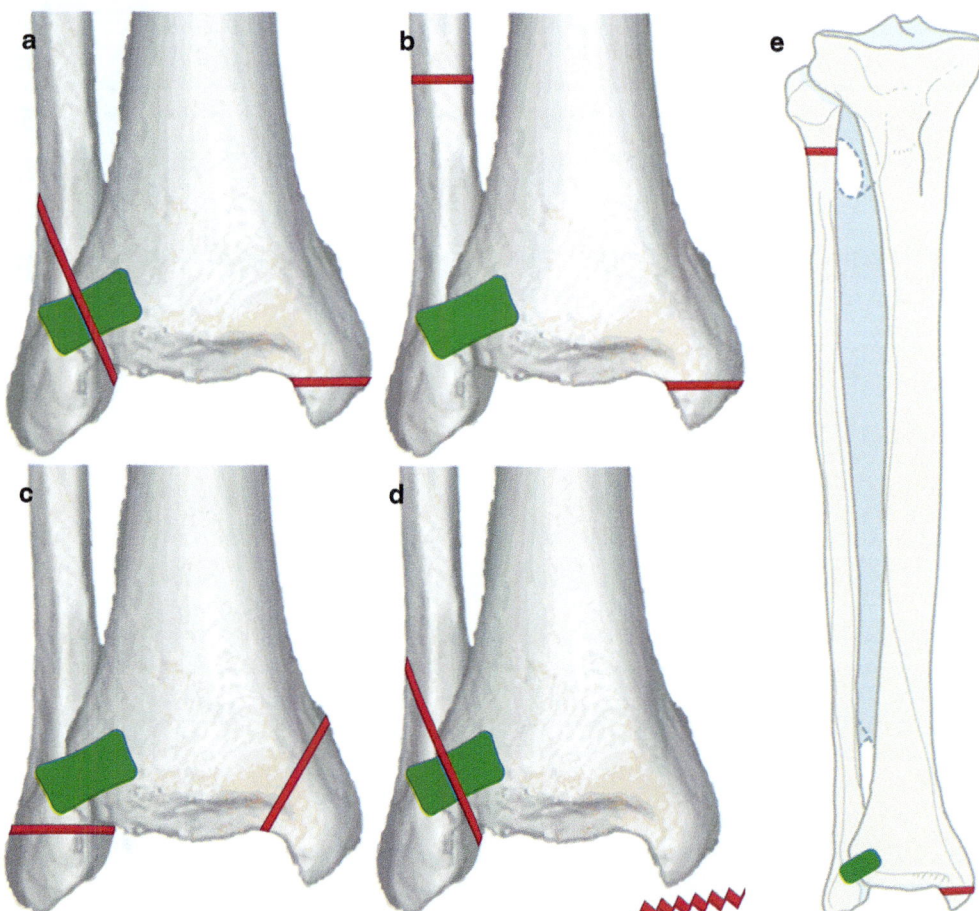

Fig. 6 (**a–e**) Bimalleolar fractures, Alnot and Duparc classification. Anterior view drawings. Interligamentary fracture (**a**), fracture above the ligament (**b**), fracture below the ligament (**c**), equivalent of a bimalleolar fracture (**d**), and Maisonneuve fracture (**e**). In green: distal tibiofibular ligaments. Red line: bone fracture. Red zigzag: medial collateral ligament rupture

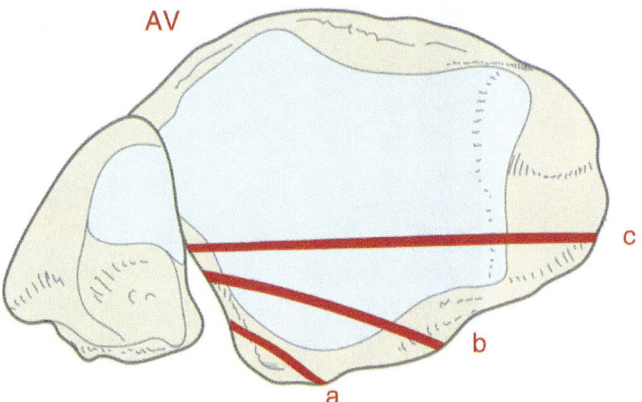

Fig. 7 Posterior tibial margin fractures related to bimalleolar fractures, seen from below. (a) Type a (extra-articular): simple avulsion of the lateral posterior tubercle. (b) Type b (articular): the most frequent, triangular fragment with lateral base. Moderate articular impact: amputation of the weight-bearing surface of the mortise <15%, the medial top does not exceed the middle part of the posterior margin. (c) Type c (articular): fragment including the totality of the posterior margin, severe articular damage with instability

Fracture of the talus [5, 9–11]:
- 1% of fractures of the whole body.
- Rare, violent hyperflexive trauma: sports and road accidents.
- 60% of the surface of the talus is articular.
  - Secondary risk of **osteoarthritis**
  - Poor vascularization, increasing the risk of **osteonecrosis** and **pseudarthrosis**
- Osteonecrosis:
  - Major risk
  - Osteosclerosis of the body of the talus
  - Occurs toward the third month and sometimes several years afterward
  - Can be responsible for a collapse of the talus
    Ankle osteoarthritis (+++)
    Flatfoot
- **Neck fracture** (Fig. 9):
  - ≈50% of talus fractures
  - Violent hyperflexive trauma

Fig. 8 (**a–d**) Pseudarthrosis on supraligamentary bimalleolar fracture, treated with immobilization. Front view of blood pool (**a**), fused sagittal slice (**b**), and frontal fused (**c**) and CT (**d**) slices. Forty-four-year-old woman, left bimalleolar fracture 9 months prior, medial malleolar pseudarthrosis discovered 3 months prior, persistent pain. Blood pool and delayed intense uptake on the fractures of the two malleoli: pseudarthrosis (arrows head). Subchondral bone suffering on the lateral part of the ankle, showing the beginnings of osteoarthritis with probable related injury to the tibiofibular syndesmosis (arrow). This case illustrates the necessity of surgical treatment with osteosynthesis for bimalleolar fractures with real tibiofibular diastasis

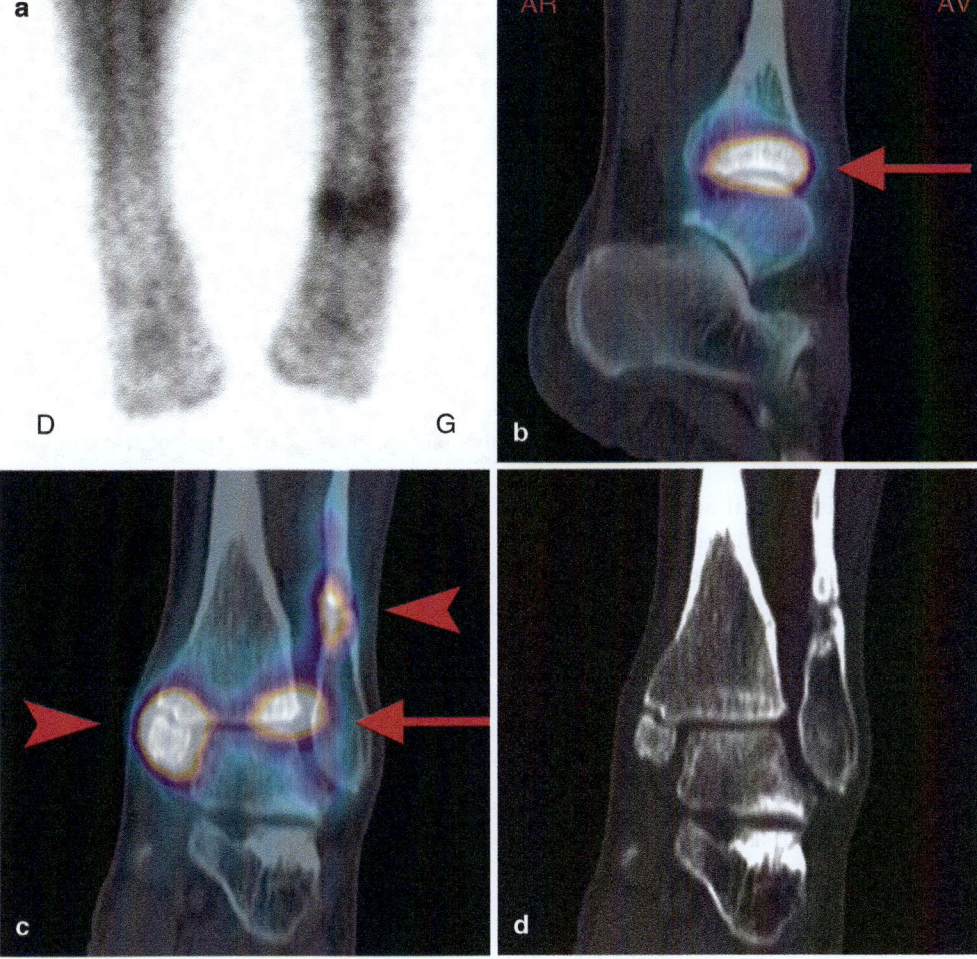

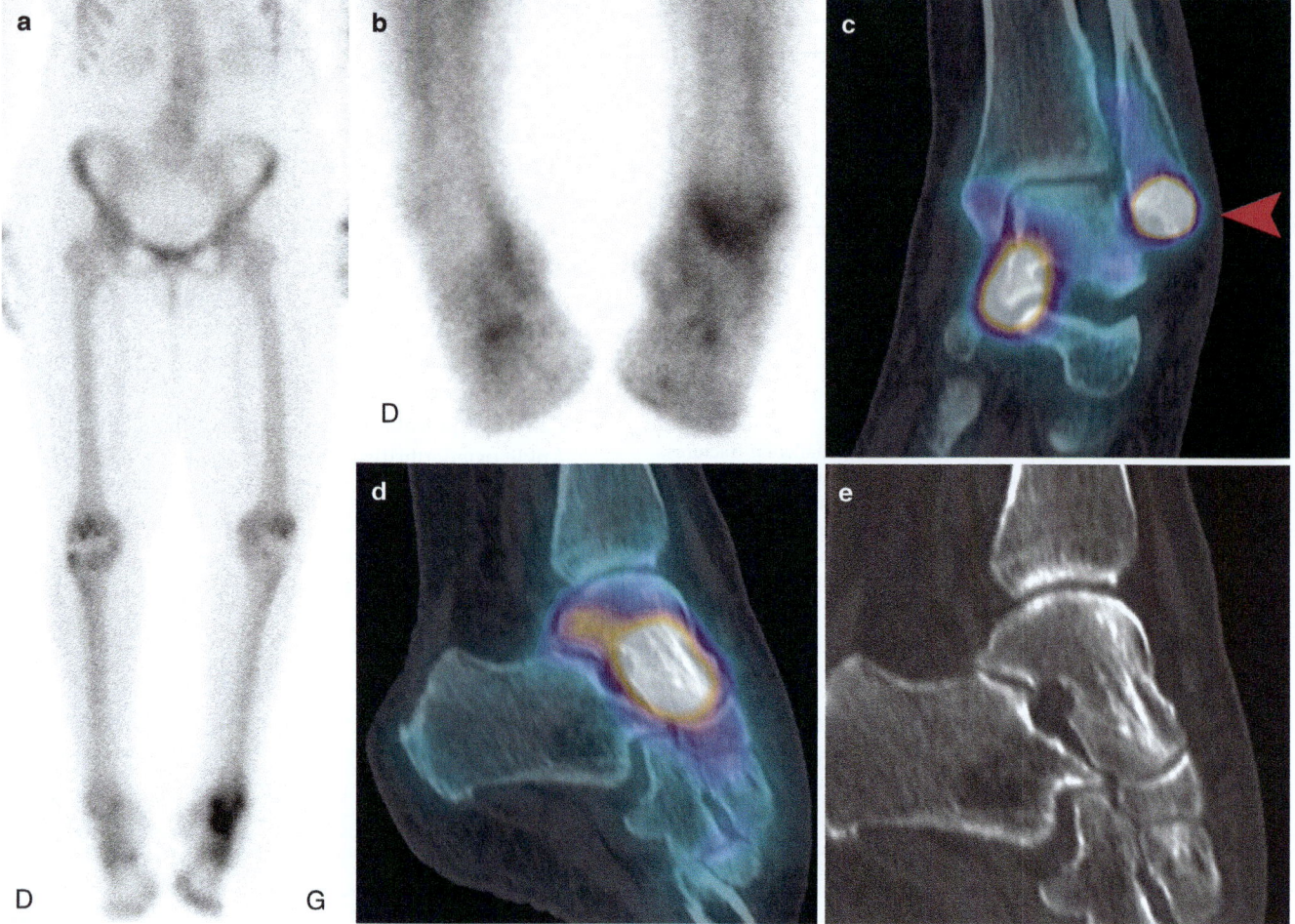

Fig. 9 (**a–e**) Recent contusion of the left talus neck. Front view of delayed (**a**) and blood pool phase (**b**), fused frontal (**c**) and sagittal (**d**) slices, sagittal CT slice (**e**). Valgus sprain 2 months prior with small bone tear on the lateral malleolus; persistent major functional infirmity. Intense uptake on bone tear (arrowhead) and discovery of intense uptake on the talus neck, without any notable anomalies in the CT, indicating a contusion without a fracture. The activity can be seen on blood pool phase, in relationship with an injury dating not more than 3 months; note the intense nature of the uptake on delayed phase

- Complications:
  Osteonecrosis of the body of the talus (+++).
    Vascularization of the body of the talus passes via the neck.
    <15% of risk if non-displaced.
    >75% if enucleation of the talus.
  Malunion (++): responsible for weight-bearing changes and secondary subtalar osteoarthritis
  Pseudarthrosis (+)
- **Fracture of the talus body:**
  - ≈20% of talus fractures
  - Fall from a high place
  - Complications:
    Osteonecrosis of the body of the talus (+++):
      <25% of risk if non-displaced
      >90% if dislocation of the talus

  Osteoarthritis (+++, 75% of cases): ankle > subtalar
  Malunion (++)
- **Fracture of the trochlea of talus:**
  - Varus sprain
  - The lateral surface of the talus crushes against the lateral malleolus or the tibia
  - Can be discovered on BS if non-displaced or if contusion without fracture line
- **Fracture of the talus head:**
  - ≈10% of talus fractures
  - Compression, falls onto the point of the feet
  - Can be discovered on BS
  - Can be associated with a navicular fracture
  - Complications:
    Osteoarthritis (++) of the talocalcaneonavicular joint
    Osteonecrosis rare as the area is well vascularized

- **Fracture of the posterior process:**
  - Primarily impacts lateral tubercle.
  - Forced extension of the ankle: compression between the tibia and the calcaneus.
  - Or forced flexion of the ankle: traction tear of the posterior talofibular ligament.
  - Differentiate from os trigonum.
- **Fracture of the lateral process:**
  - Snowboard trauma (+++)
  - Delay in diagnosis ≈ 70%, can be discovered on BS
  - Complications:
    Osteonecrosis and pseudarthrosis (not well vascularized)
    Subtalar osteoarthritis
    Malunion: conflict with the fibula

Fracture of the calcaneus [9–11]:
- 1–2% of fractures of the whole body
- 60% of fractures of the tarsus
- **Fracture of the body:**
  - Fall from height onto heels
  - Serious fractures: often complex, with depressions, very often through the posterior talar articular surface
  - Complications:
    Secondary subtalar osteoarthritis (+++), even in the event of well-treated fracture
- **Fracture of the dorsal part of the anterior process** [11] (Fig. 10):
  - Fracture or tear by traction on the bifurcate ligament
  - Can be seen on BS

Fracture of the navicular [9]:
- Rare
- Major injury, often associated with other fractures
- **Fracture of the body:**
  - Serious
  - Complications:
    Osteonecrosis and pseudarthrosis (Fig. 11)
    Architectural modification of the medial longitudinal arch
- **Avulsion of the tuberosity:**
  - Partial tear of the tibialis posterior tendon

Fracture of the cuboid [9]:
- Rare, exceptionally isolated

Dislocation of transverse tarsal joint [9]:
- Rare, major injury

Tarsometatarsal dislocation [9]:
- Rather rare
- Injury:
  - Severe
  - Or moderate: dislocation can pass unnoticed.
- Possible related bone injuries, at the level of the articulation:
  - Laterodistal angle of the cuboid (+)
  - Base of M1
- Complications:
  - Mechanical tarsometatarsal pain
  - Architectural disorders with metatarsalgia

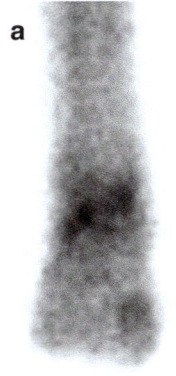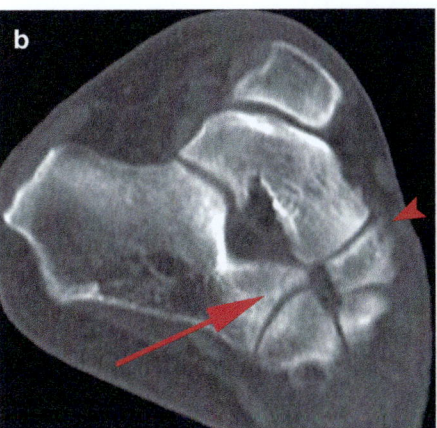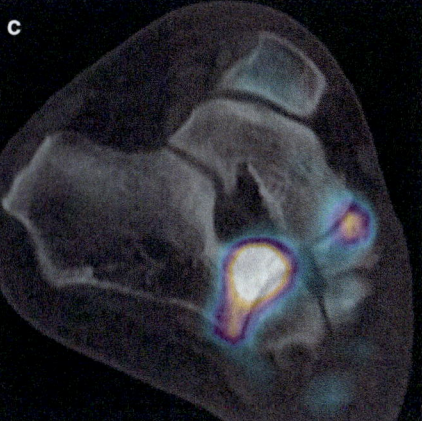

Fig. 10 (**a–c**) Recent fracture of the dorsal part of the anterior process of calcaneus (arrow) and small dorsal proximal navicular bone tear (arrowhead) in a sprain of the transverse tarsal joint. Front view of blood pool phase (**a**), oblique sagittal CT (**b**), and fused (**c**) slices. Persistent pain after injury of the right foot 1 month prior: note the focused intense uptake visible on blood pool phase and the distribution of CT and scintigraphic anomalies in the dorsal part of the transverse tarsal joint. The fracture of the dorsal part of the anterior process shows damage to the bifurcate ligament, and the bone tear on the upper edge of the navicular shows that the talonavicular ligament has been damaged

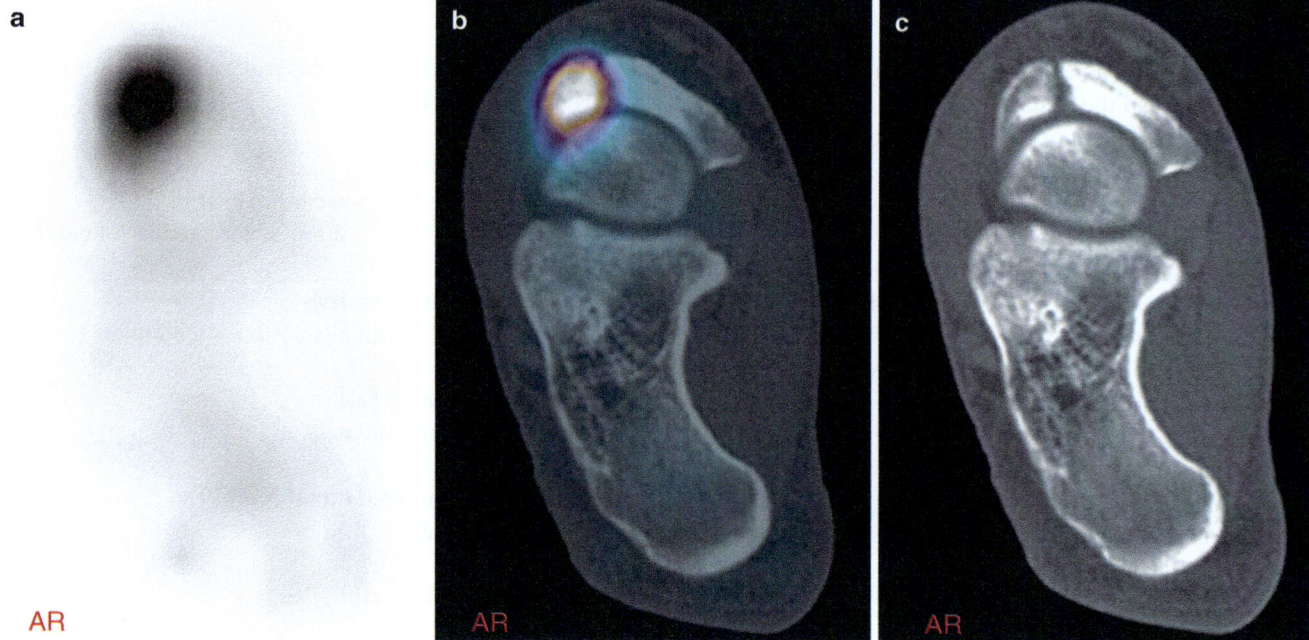

Fig. 11 (**a–c**) Sequelae of fracture of the body of the navicular. Axial scintigraphic (**a**), fused (**b**), and CT (**c**) slices. Possible osteonecrosis, but one cannot formally eliminate pseudarthrosis

Box 3
Fractures of the ankle and foot that can be discovered on bone scan:

- Bimalleolar:
  - Maisonneuve Fx
- Distal tibial epiphysis:
  - Posterior margin Fx
- Talus:
  - Trochlea Fx
  - Head Fx
  - Lateral process Fx
- Calcaneus:
  - Dorsal part of the anterior process Fx

Stress Fractures

Predisposition:

- Athletes/military training: intensification and/or changes in training
- Woman overtraining with the triad: amenorrhea, osteoporosis, and eating disorders with low BMI
- Nonathletes: prolonged unusual effort (mountain hiking, etc.)

Past medical history:
- Stress fractures (SFx)

Frequency [12–14]:
- **Frequent**, approximately 10% of sports-related injuries
- Localization in athletes (cf. following page)
  - Tibia (50%)
  - Tarsus (25%):
    Posterior tarsus: talus, calcaneus
    Anterior tarsus: navicular (8%)
      cuboid (rare)
      cuneiform (rare)
  - Metatarsals (10%)
  - Femur (8%)
  - Fibula (5%)
  - Sesamoid (1%)

Mechanism [15, 16]:
- The fracture occurs outside of any specific trauma when there is a discrepancy between bone resistance and the stress put upon it. In the bone's attempt to adapt, bone remodeling increases, with the initial consequence being excess resorption, which boosts short-term fracture risk [13].

Types [15]:
Different types of bones are prone to different types of fractures:

- Cortical fracture: impacts the metatarsals (especially the neck of M2 and M3), +/− distal extremities of the tibia and fibula
- Spongy fracture: impacts the tarsal bones, the base and head of the metatarsals, and the distal extremities of the tibia and fibula
- Cortico-spongy fracture: corresponds to an advanced stage of a cortical or spongy fracture and combines a fracture of the spongy bone and the adjacent cortex

Interview:
- Mechanical pain:
  - Increasing gradually in intensity
  - Occurring earlier and earlier during effort
  - Calmed by the rest
- Concept of uncommon effort

Clinical examination:
- Precise localized pain
- +/− localized swelling

Paraclinical examination [15, 17]:
- X-ray: delayed visibility of SFx, 10–15 days after the beginning of the clinical symptoms
- CT: delayed visibility of SFx; fracture line perpendicular to the bone's lines of force, periosteal apposition
- MRI: early visibility of SFx; edema of the spongy bone and soft parts

Differential [16]:
- Depends on the localization:
  - Tendinopathy
  - Nerve entrapment
  - Degenerative or inflammatory arthropathy

Classification:
- Pre-fracture:
  - Early stage
  - Reversible by removing stress
  - Pain
  - Spongy contusion
- Fracture:
  - Can be avoided if stress removed early on
  - Pain
  - Cortical fracture line, periosteal apposition

Evolution:
- Risk of **pseudarthrosis**

Treatment [14, 16]:
- **Activity modification**
- If SFx located at a spot with no risk of pseudarthrosis:
  - Partial stress relief, allowing painless activity
  - For 4–6 weeks
- In SFX located at a spot at risk of pseudarthrosis:
  - Orthopedic consultation
  - Complete stress relief or surgery

Discussion:

- MRI and BS are very useful for the diagnosis of SFx and show both good Se and good Sp [18].
- Studies try to evaluate the prognostic contribution of these techniques in the treatment of SFx and the time before resuming activities, particularly for high-level athletes.
- A study of 84 athletes with suspected SFx evaluated the interest of BS (without SPECT-CT). There were 50 SFx in the end: the BS had a Se of 97% and a Sp of 67%. Ranked by severity as seen on the BS, the SFx of low rank (weak and irregular uptake) had an average healing time of 81 days, whereas the higher-ranking SFx (strong and well-delimited uptake) took longer to heal—147 days on average [19].
- A retrospective study by the same team focused on 52 high-level athletes, studying the interest of the functional imagery for predicting the time needed before resuming sport after SFx. They used BS (without SPECT-CT) and MRI to establish a rank of severity from low rank (weak and irregular uptake in BS/osseous edema on STIR even in T2 with the MRI) to high rank (strong and well-delimited uptake in BS/osseous edema in T1 and T2 with the MRI). They then combined these two ranks of severity from the imagery with the risk of pseudarthrosis based on the topography of the SFx (low risk and high risk of pseudarthrosis) to obtain four groups. MRI and BS severity ranks nearly all matched ($k > 0.8$). In the event of SFx in sites with a high risk of pseudarthrosis, whatever the rank in imagery, and in the event of SFx on sites at low risk of pseudarthrosis but of high rank in imagery, the time before resuming activities was long (approximately 130–150 days). In the event of SFx at a spot with low risk of pseudarthrosis and low rank in imagery, the time before resuming activities was shorter (approximately 60 days) [18].
- On the contrary, another retrospective study on 40 patients suffering from tibial SFx with low risk of pseudarthrosis found that the extent and the intensity of uptake on BS (without SPECT-CT) were not predictive of healing time (which was 50 days on average) [20].

Box 4

Stress fractures at risk of pseudarthrosis (related to bone sites in tension (and not in compression) or with little vascularization) [14]:

- Sesamoids
- Navicular
- Talus: neck
- Base of the fifth metatarsal
- Base of the second metatarsal
- Tibia: medial malleolus and anterior cortex
- Femur: superior lateral fracture of the femoral neck

Stress Fractures: Common Localization

Tibia [12]**:** The most frequent localization (Figs. 12 and 13):
- **Longitudinal fracture of the inferior 1/3 of the tibia:**
  - Athletes
  - Cortical fracture
  - Vertical cortical fracture line
  - Differentiate from posteromedial tibial periostitis (shin splints) [16] (Fig. 14)
- **Transverse fracture of the tibial metaphysis:**
  - Spongy fracture

- **Fracture of the medial malleolus:**
  - Athletes
  - Spongy fracture
  - At the junction between the tibial pilon and the malleolus
  - Risk of pseudarthrosis

Talus [12] (excluding osteochondral lesions of the talus) (Fig. 15):
- **Subchondral fracture**:
  - Can impact the dome, head, and lower posterior surface (Fig. 16)
  - Spongy fracture

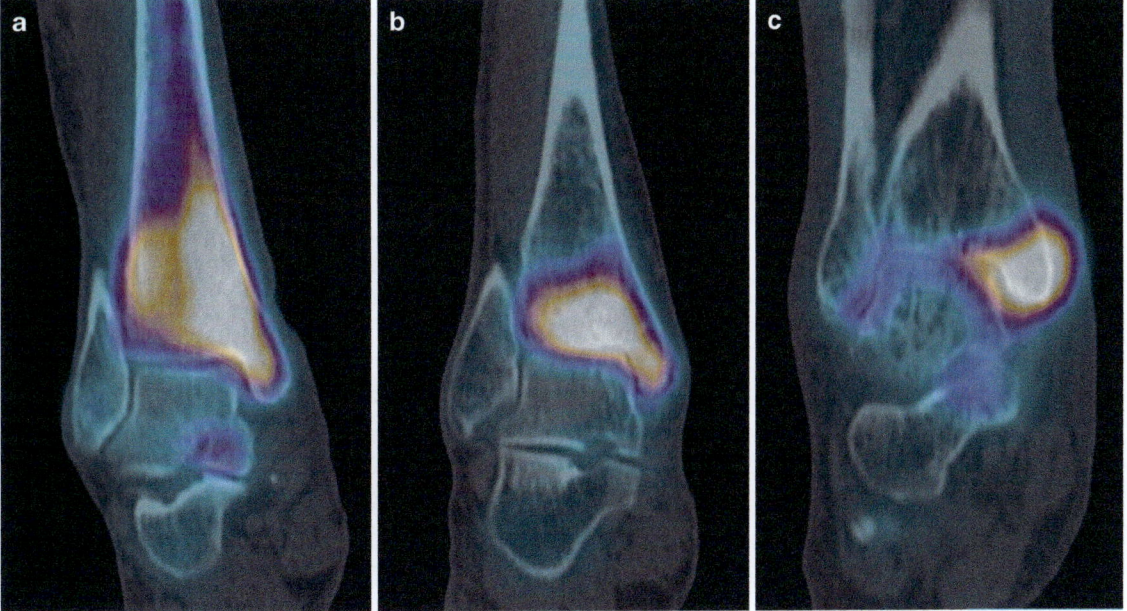

Fig. 12 (**a–c**) Tibial stress fractures, fused frontal slices: longitudinal fracture of the inferior third of the tibia (**a**), transverse fracture of the tibial metaphysis (**b**), and fracture of the medial malleolus (**c**)

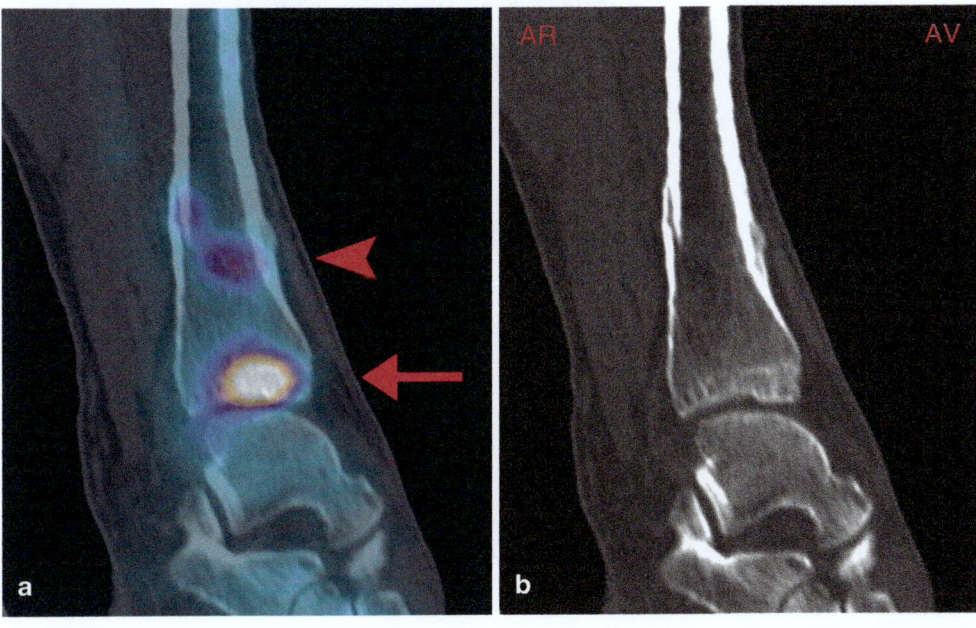

Fig. 13 (**a** and **b**) Stress fracture of the distal epiphysis of the tibia, fused (**a**) and CT (**b**) sagittal slices. Prior fracture of the lower part of the tibial diaphysis (arrowhead). Good consolidation but with slight anterior angulation of the distal fragment, responsible for a modification of weight bearing, resulting in an underlying stress fracture (arrow)

Fig. 14 (a–c) Bilateral tibial periostitis, posterior view of WB (a), fused transverse (b) and frontal slices (c). Thirty-year-old patient practicing football: note the topography of activity around the periosteum, corresponding to the flexor digitorum longus insertion zone

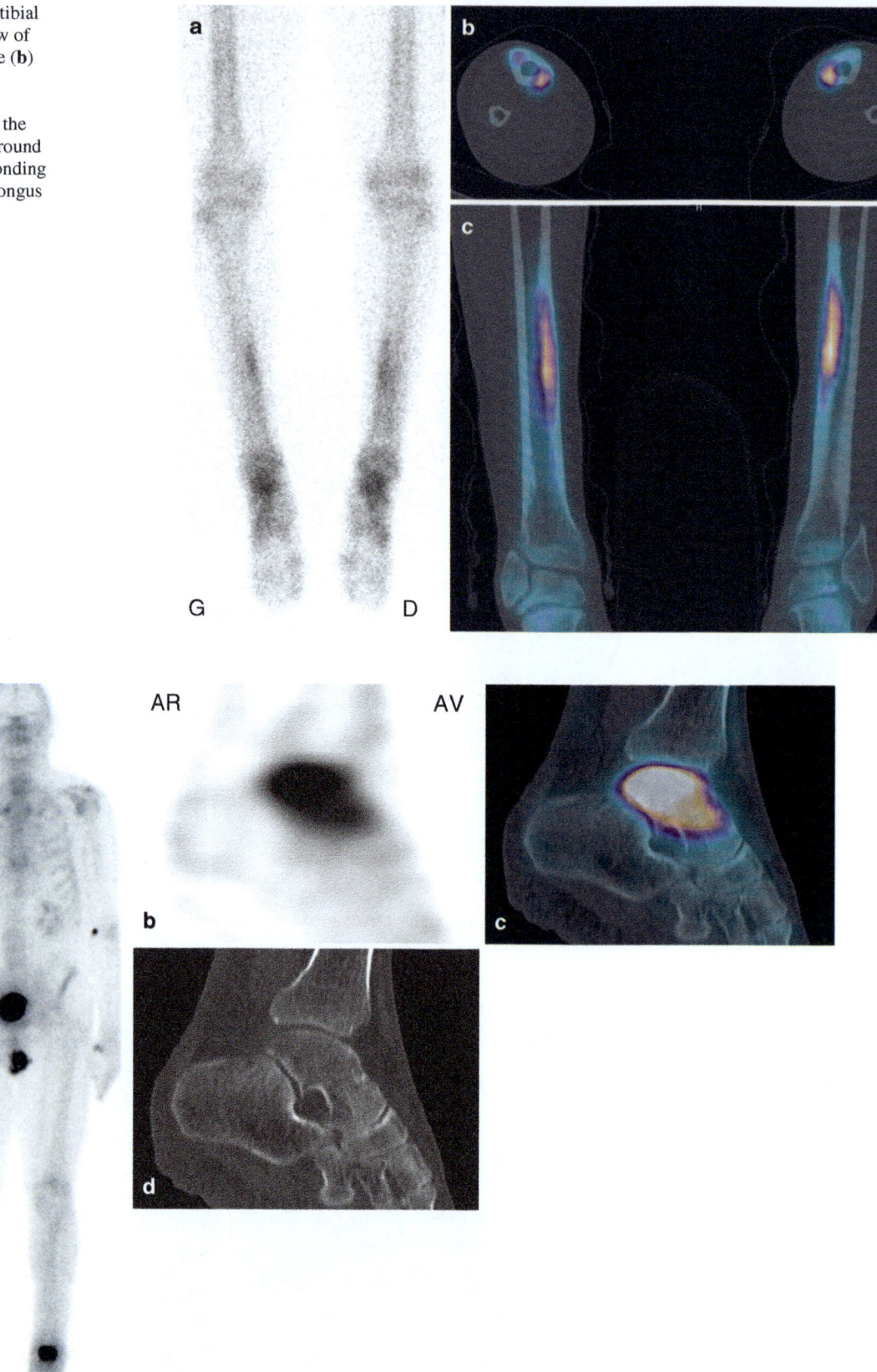

Fig. 15 (a–d) Stress fracture of the body of the left talus. Anterior view of WB (a), scintigraphic (b), fused (c), and CT (d) sagittal slices. Pain in left foot for the past 3 months: context of right limp-ing due to coxarthrosis (arrowhead), involving a shift in weight bearing onto the lower left limb. Note intense uptake without CT injury

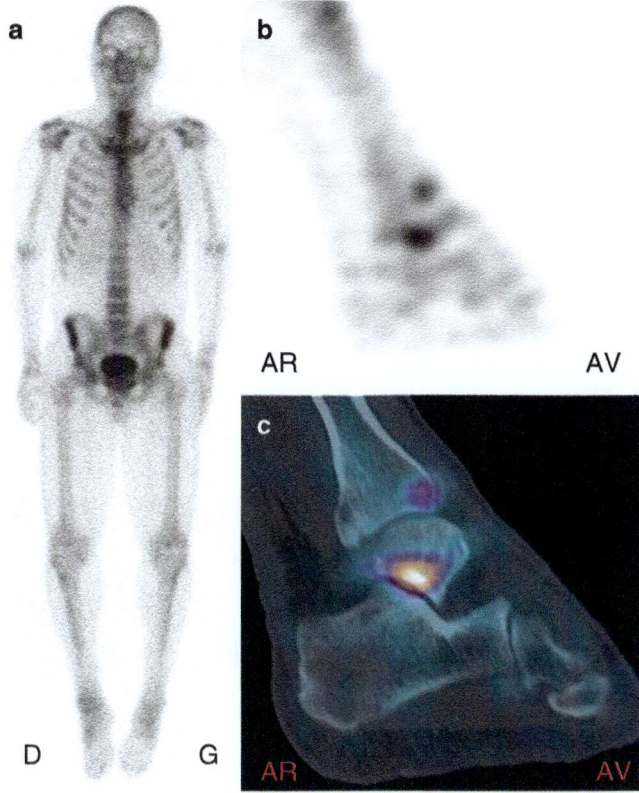

Fig. 16 (**a–c**) Subchondral stress fracture of the lower posterior surface of the right talus. Anterior view of WB (**a**), scintigraphic slices (**b**) and fused images (**c**). High-level athlete (marathon runner), right ankle discomfort for approximately 2 years; no explanation found on the arthro-CT carried out 2 months prior: discrete subchondral uptake on the talar side of the subtalar joint, without anomalies seen on the CT and nearly invisible on the WB scan. The same aspect can be seen on the left foot, which is even more moderate (not shown). Note the nearly insignificant activity on the anterior tibial distal epiphysis, which could result from an anterior ankle impingement

- **Fracture of the lateral process**:
  - Cortico-spongy fracture
  - Athletes (running)
- **Fracture of the lateral posterior process**:
  - Athletes in hyperextension (dance)
  - Related to a chronic impingement of the process wedged between the tibia and the calcaneus

Calcaneus [12]:
- **Fracture of the tuberosity (+++)** (Fig. 17):
  - Posterior spongy bone fracture
  - Athletes (running)
  - Postmenopause overweight women
  - Vertical line:
    Roughly parallel to the posterior cortical
    Perpendicular to the main spongy trabecula

- **Fracture of the anterior process**
- **Fracture of the sustentaculum tali**

Metatarsals [12]: frequent (running, soldiers), predominantly on M2 and M3
- **Fracture of the neck**:
  - Most frequent
  - Cortical fracture
- **Fracture of the base of M2** (Fig. 18):
  - Cortico-spongy fracture
  - Risk of pseudarthrosis
  - Dancers (points)
- **Fracture of the base of M5** [13]:
  - Approximately 1.5 cm in front of the tuberosity of M5
    Risk of pseudarthrosis
    Must differentiate from the more frequent avulsion fracture of the tuberosity, which is not at risk of pseudarthrosis
- **Fracture of a metatarsal head**:
  - Rare

Femur [13, 14]:
- Athletes, in particular female (running, track and field), soldiers
- **Neck fracture**:
  - Superior-lateral: mechanism in tension, worse prognosis (risk of complete fracture, then displacement, then osteonecrosis or pseudarthrosis)
  - Inferior-medial: mechanism in compression
- **Diaphysis fracture**:
  - Medial, at the 1/3 proximal-1/3 medial junction

Fibula [13]:
- Athletes (running)
- Transverse line, a little above the tibiofibular syndesmosis

Navicular [12, 17]:
- Cortical fracture.
- Athletes (track and field, running, jumping, etc.).
- Sagittal line, proximal and dorsal on medial 1/3 of the navicular bone.
- Complications include complete fracture, in the least vascularized area of the bone, with risk of osteonecrosis.

Sesamoid [12, 15]:
- Impacts the medial hallux sesamoid (+++)
- Athletes (gymnasts, ballerinas)
- Woman wearing high heels
- Risk of osteonecrosis

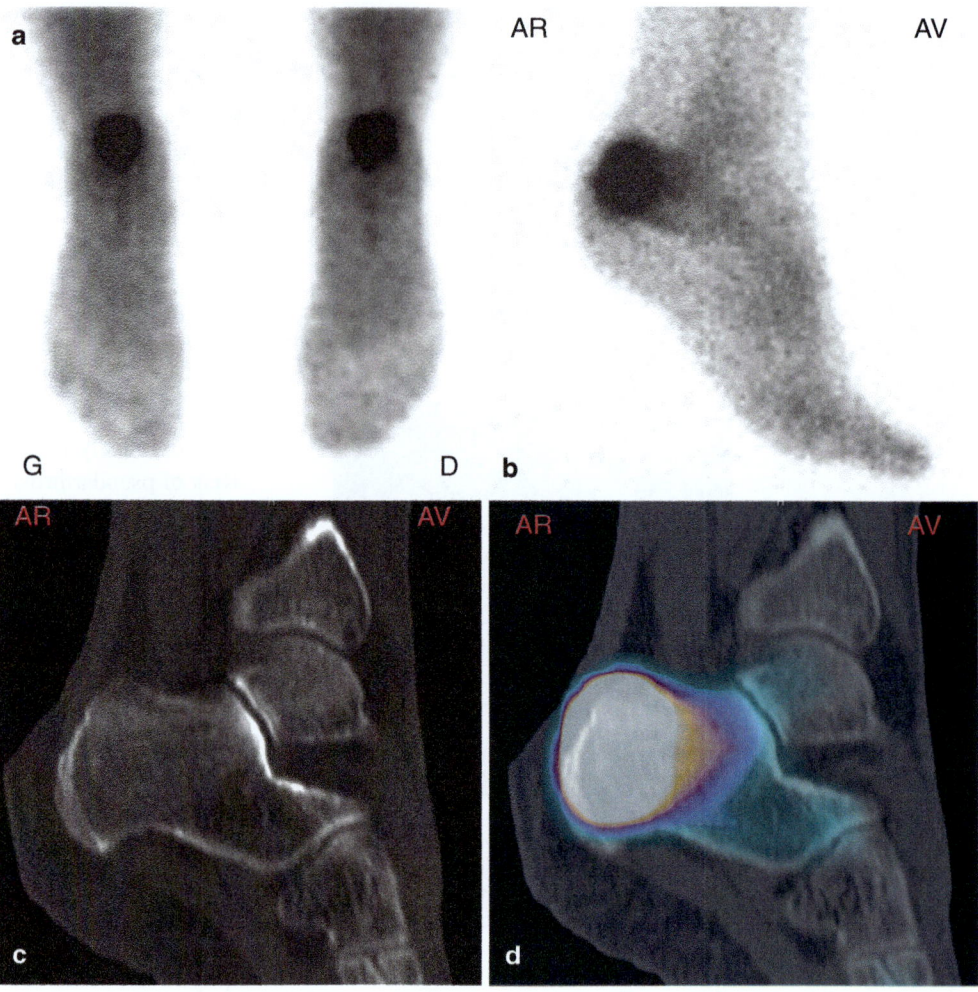

Fig. 17 (**a–d**) Bilateral stress fracture of the calcaneus tuberosity, plantar blood pool phase (**a**), delayed side-view image (**b**), sagittal CT (**c**), and fused (**d**) slices. Fifty-four-year-old patient, with known osteoporosis, recent pain after walking for a day and half

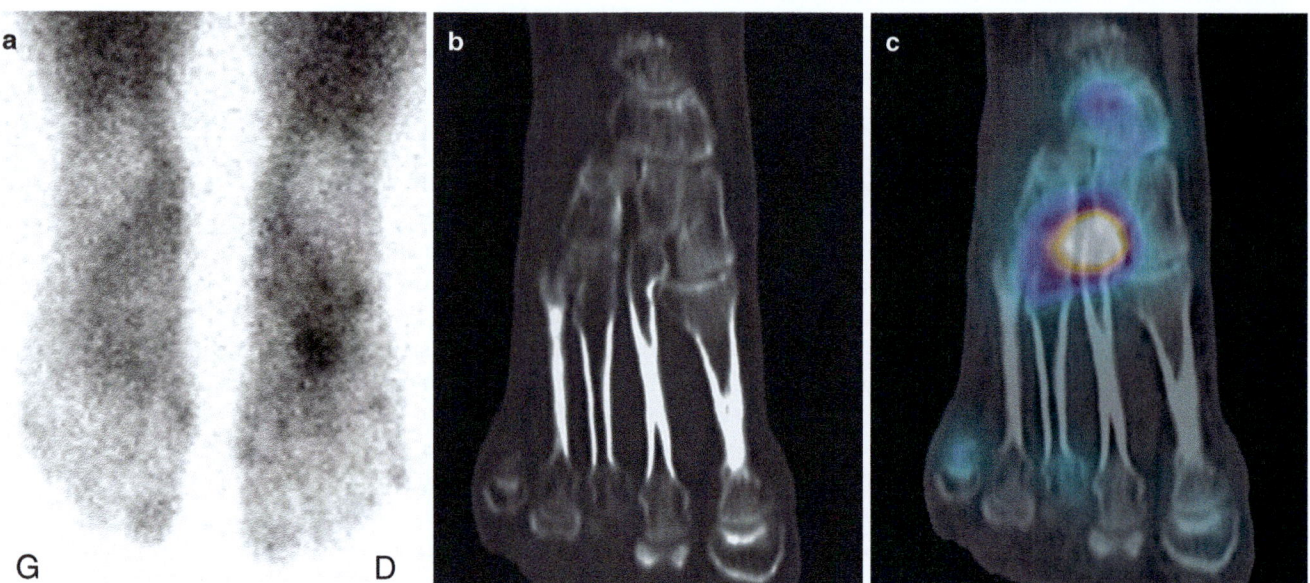

Fig. 18 (**a–c**) Stress fracture of the right M2 base, plantar blood pool phase (**a**), transverse CT (**b**), and fused (**c**) slices. The base of M2 is not very mobile because it is wedged in the mortise produced by the three cuneiform bones, whereas the other part of M2 is more mobile. This localization runs the risk of pseudarthrosis and usually requires immobilization or even osteosynthesis

Osteochondral Lesions of the Talus (OLT) (aka Osteochondritis Dissecans of the Talus or Talar Osteochondral Lesion)

Predisposition:
- Man > woman (M/F = 3/2)
- Any age, especially between 20 and 50 years

Past medical history [21]:
- **Trauma:**
  - In ≈ 95% of lateral OLT
  - In ≈ 65% of medial OLT [22]

Frequency [21]:
- Probably underestimated.
- Incidence = 9 cases per 100,000 person-years.
- Found in ≈ 6% of ankle sprains.
- Medial OLT is a little more frequent than lateral OLT (Fig. 19).

Mechanism:
- *If traumatic causes*: the edge of the talus dome impacting the ankle mortise.
  - Lateral edge more often involved than the medial edge.
- *In the absence of traumatic cause*: process of partial necrosis (vascular, hormonal, toxic, hereditary, etc., etiology) (Fig. 20)

Types:
- **Acute**: in the 6 weeks following an injury
- **Chronic**: most frequent, with or without traumatic history

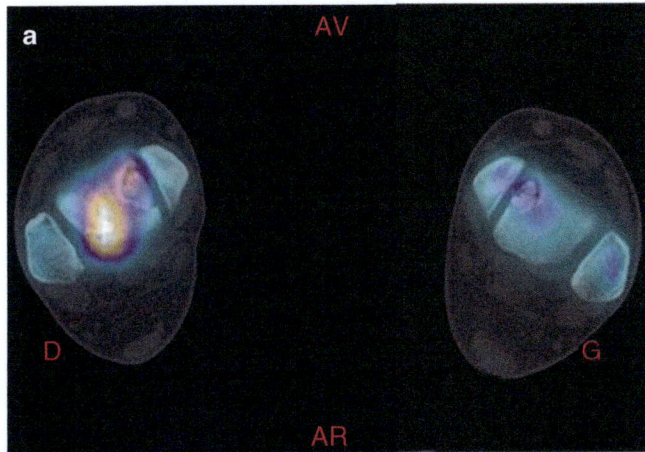

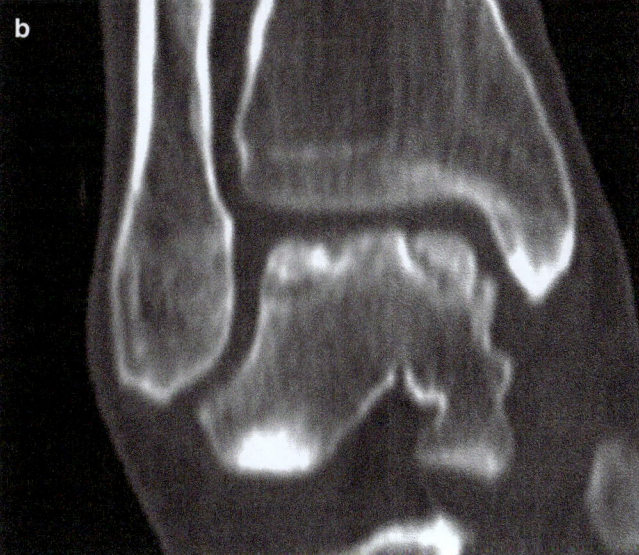

Fig. 20 (**a** and **b**) Bilateral OLT secondary to cortisone treatment, transverse fused (**a**) and frontal CT (**b**) slices of the right foot. Forty-six-year-old man, treated with cortisone for several years for Behcet and Crohn disease. Prior osteonecrosis of the medial left femur condyle 6 years before. Pain in the sacroiliac joints (normal bone scan, not shown) and moderate right ankle discomfort, without prior trauma: note the evolutive partial necrosis process on the dome of the right talus (medial and lateral) and the lesser-evolutive necrosis on the dome of the left talus (medial)

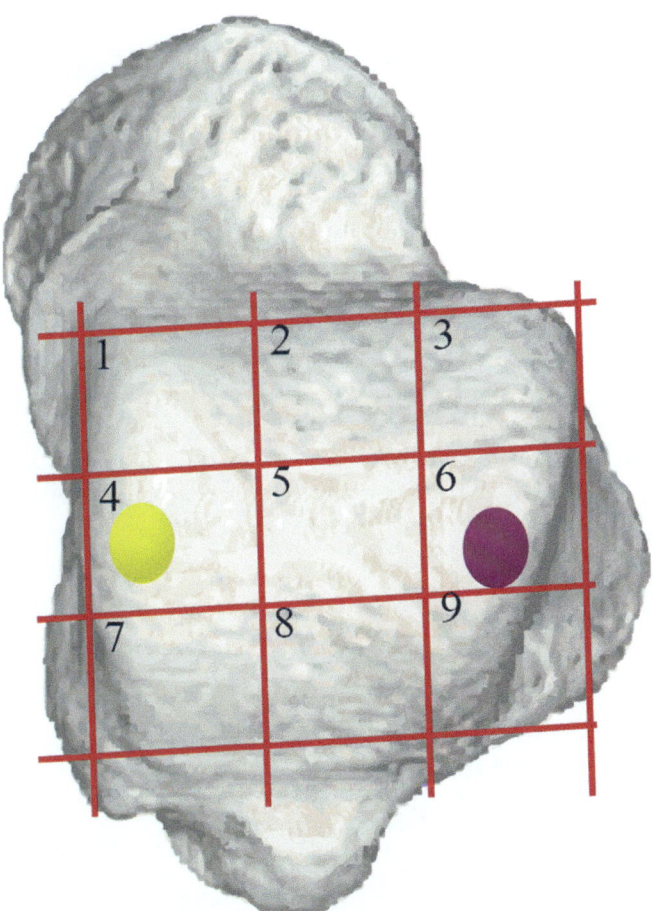

Fig. 19 OLT localization: Nine-grid scheme based on Elias et al. Zones 4 (medial and mid, in yellow) and 6 (lateral and mid, in purple) are most frequently impacted: approximately 55% and 25% of the lesions, respectively

Interview and clinical examination:

- Nonspecific
- Ankle pain:
  - Mechanical
  - With mobilization
- Swelling, cracking
- +/−stiffness

Paraclinical examination [21]:

- X-ray:
  - Can be normal
  - Can show a notch or a subchondral geode
- CT (very specific):
  - To visualize the bone structure
  - To assess surface/depth of the OLT, the presence of a geode
- Artho-CT (+++): additional examination of the cartilage
- MRI (very sensitive):
  - To evaluate the cartilage, visualize subchondral edema.

Differential [16]:

- All the causes of atypical or chronic ankle pain (Fig. 21).
- Paraclinical examinations enable a confirmation of the diagnosis.

Classification [21]:

- **Lateral OLT** (Fig. 22):
  - Trauma etiology (+++)
  - Classically the anterior and medial parts
  - Width > depth
  - Blurred edges

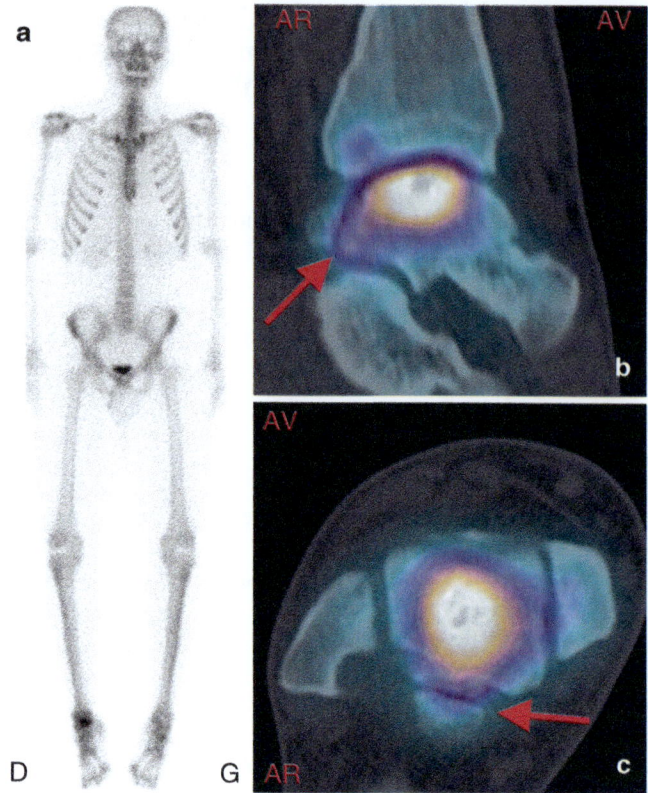

Fig. 21 (**a–c**) Median OLT, anterior view of WB (**a**), fused sagittal (**b**) and transverse (**c**) slices. Twenty-two-year-old man, persistent right ankle pain: suspicion of posterior conflict. No uptake anomaly on the synchondrosis between the lateral tubercle of the talus and the os trigonum (arrow). Discovery of an isolated very evolutive median OLT

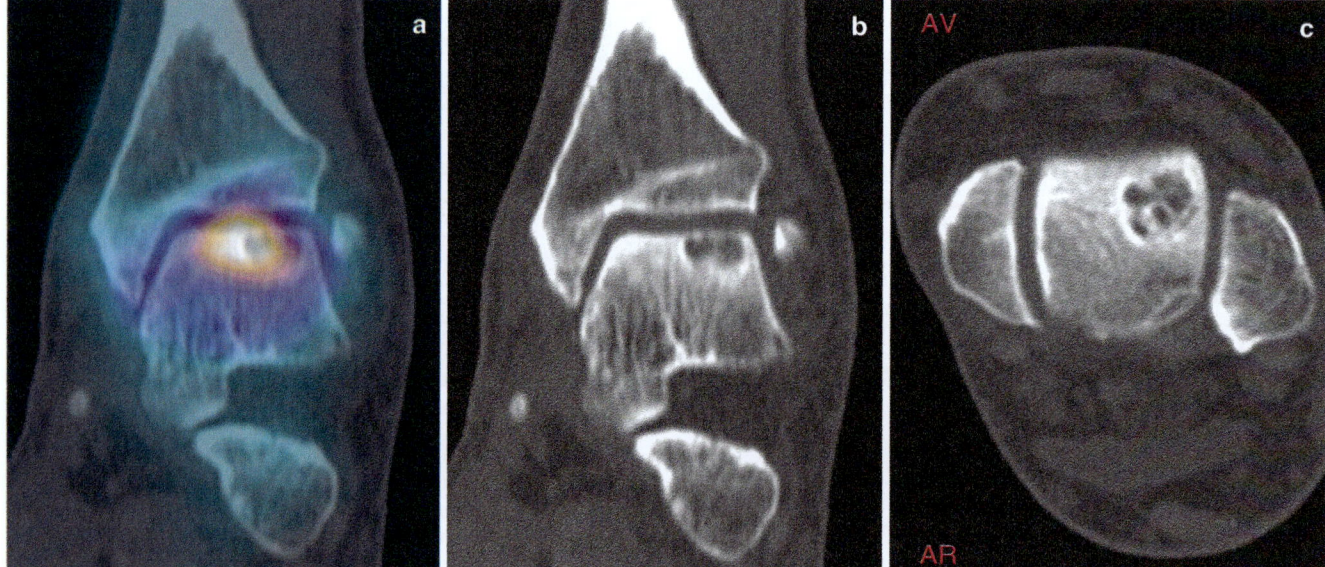

Fig. 22 (**a–c**) Known anterolateral OLT in a 60-year-old man, prior repeated sprains. Frontal fused (**a**) and CT (**b**) slices, transverse CT slice (**c**). Scintigraphic evaluation: evolutive OLT, without any other lesion. Note the lesion is broader rather than high and the presence of subchondral geodes

- **Medial OLT**:
  - Trauma etiology (+++)
  - Classically the posterior part
  - Depth > width
  - Sharp edges

Evolution [21]:

- Natural evolution: persistent pain, symptomatic osteoarthritis (1% of the patients)
- Evolution under treatment: improvement of the symptoms, frequent return to sports (85% of the patients) [22]
- Factors of poor prognosis: size of lesion >1.5 cm^2, displaced fragment

Principle of treatment [21]:

- Care depends on the size, the stability and the viability of the lesion, and the extent of articular cartilage damage.
- **Acute OLT**: possible quick osteosynthesis if viable fragment.
- **Chronic OLT**: not urgent.
  - *Conservative Tx*: for the small undetached lesions [23], considered if age >55 years.
    Rest +/− immobilization and NSAIDs
    Success rate <50%
  - *Surgical Tx* (++): frequently requires malleolus osteotomy in view of accessing the zone of the operation. Debridement and stimulation of bone marrow (+++)
    +/− cartilaginous autograft
    +/− osteocartilaginous allograft

Discussion:

- Information collected from a bone SPECT/CT can change OLT care in 50% of the cases compared to the MRI alone: the subchondral uptake is almost always smaller than the medullary edema zone visualized with the MRI (which thus overestimates the lesions). The authors recommend the analysis of both MRI and bone SPECT/CT for OLT [24]. There are few studies, but the experience seems to show that BS is more specific than MRI for OLT exams: In the absence of uptake on the BS, the OLT is not responsible for the patient's pain [25].
- A study of 15 OLT cases showed that there is a major correlation between pain and uptake seen on SPECT/CT [26]. In a study on 22 OLT cases, the authors estimated that the SPECT/CT enabled selection of which cases to operate as a result of uptake, to prepare the operation based on the depth of uptake, and led to discovery of other lesions explaining the symptoms when there was no OLT uptake [27].
- A team which had worked on SPECT/CT arthrography of the wrist [28] showed the feasibility of bone SPECT/CT associated with the injection of the contrast medium in the ankle, particularly in OLT and ankle osteoarthritis diagnosis [29].

Box 5

In the event of even moderate uptake in the ankle on a whole-body bone scintigraphy, one should carry out bone SPECT/CT looking for OLT if:

- The patient is young (uptake does not correspond to osteoarthritis).
- And there is ankle pain/discomfort.
- And there has been prior ankle trauma.

Box 6
Classifications
There are many OLT classifications. We will describe the FOG and Ferkel systems, which are the most used.

- **FOG classification** (1995, Dore and Rosset) (Fig. 23):
  - Based on X-ray and CT images of the OLT
  - Can be used in SPECT/CT

    F form (fractures): bone fragment with no modification of the underlying bone matrix. Can be recent or old. Constant traumatic history

    O form (osteonecrosis): sequestrum with underlying condensation and geodes. Rare traumatic history

    G form (geode, bone cyst): absence of free fragment or sequestrum. Subchondral geode(s). Frequent history of traumatic or microtraumatic injuries

- **Ferkel classification** (1993):
  - Based on arthro-CT scan aspect of the OLT
  - Takes into account the state of the cartilage, which conditions both Tx and prognosis
  - Cannot be used in SPECT/CT

    Stage I: intact articular surface, subchondral geode

    Stage IIa: open cartilage, subchondral geode

    Stage IIb: open cartilage, non-displaced fragment

    Stage III: open cartilage, non-displaced fragment, subchondral geode

    Stade IV: displaced fragment

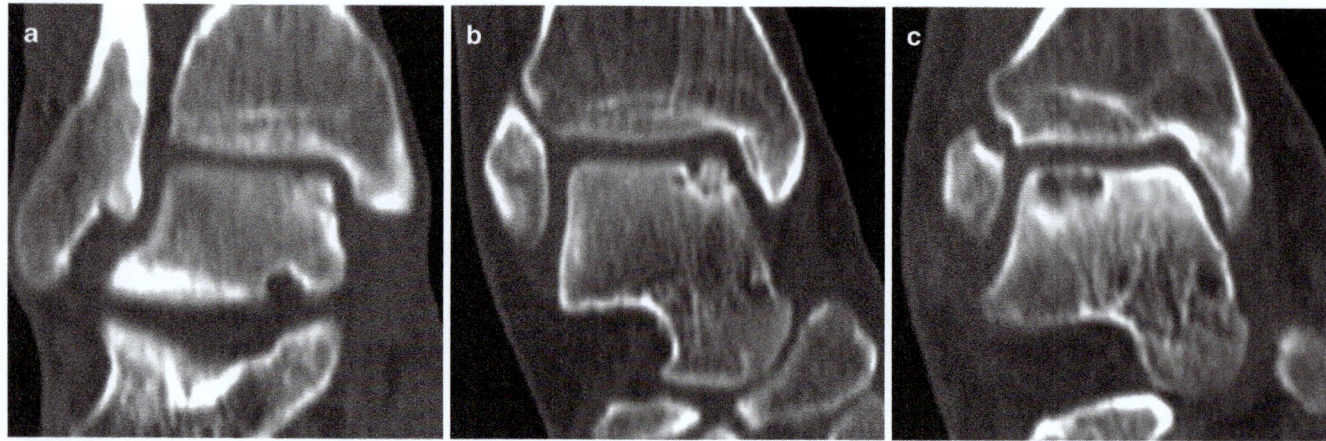

Fig. 23 (**a–c**) FOG OLT classification, frontal CT slices (**a–c**). F form as fracture (**a**), O form as osteonecrosis (**b**), and G form as geode (**c**)

Anterior Ankle Impingement

Predisposition:
- **Athletes**: with movements of forced ankle flexion
- Football players (++), dancers, gymnasts, runners

Past medical history: NR
Frequency:
- Frequent in football players and dancers

Mechanism [12, 30]:
- Repeated ankle flexions lead to microinjuries of the anterior distal tibial epiphysis and the dorsal part of the neck of talus. The microinjuries lead to hemorrhages of the periosteum with neoformation of bony spurs: During ankle flexion, soft tissues get stuck between the spurs and cause painful limitations.

Types: NR
Interview and clinical examination:
- Ankle pain:
  - Chronic
  - Anterior
  - Increased with ankle flexion
  - With palpation of the anterior part of ankle joint

Paraclinical examination [12]:
- **X-rays (+++):**
  - **Bony spurs**, **mirrored** on the anterior portion of the distal tibial epiphysis and on the dorsal part of the neck of talus (Fig. 24)
- Arthro-CT:
  - Bone spurs.
  - Anterior synovitis.
  - Search for related ankle cartilaginous lesion.
  - Assess the joint cavity prior to arthroscopy.
- Arthro-MRI:
  - Bone spurs.
  - Anterior synovitis.
  - Spongy edema in the impingement zones.
  - Look for related ankle osteochondral lesions.

Differential:
- Related ankle osteochondral lesions

Classification [30]:
- Scranton and Mcdermott: based on the degree of osteophyte (spur) formation
- Van Dijk system: based on the presence of osteophytes and ankle osteoarthritis on X-rays

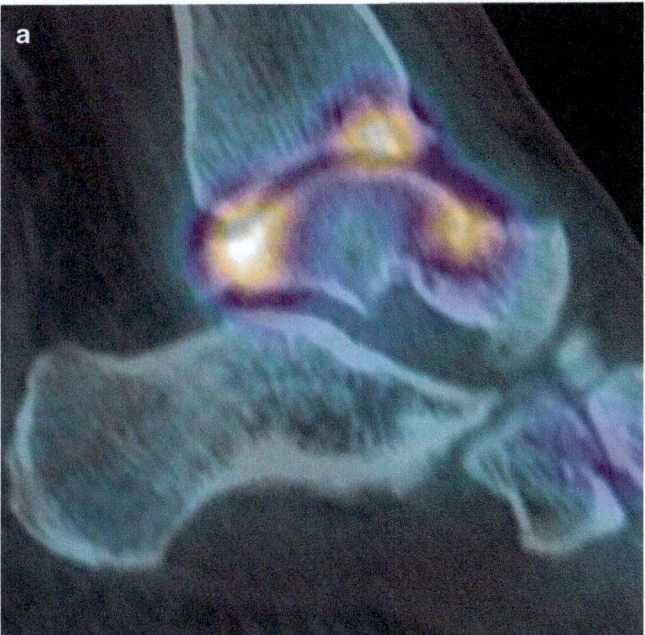

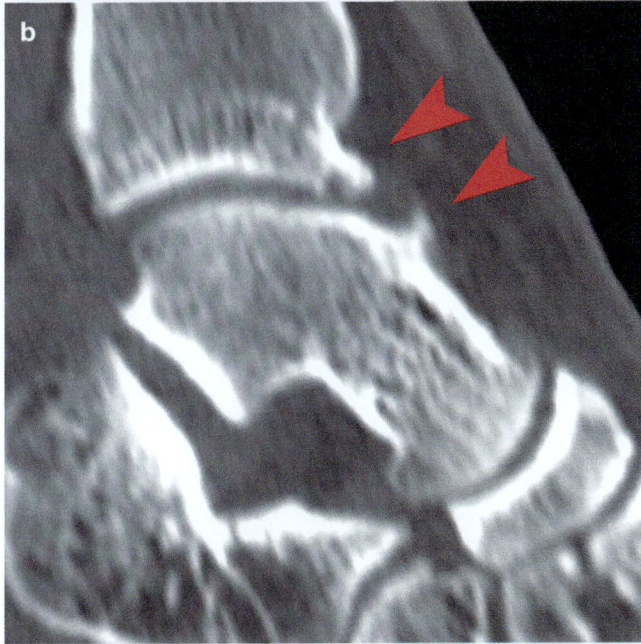

Fig. 24 (**a** and **b**) Anterior and posterior impingement, fused sagittal slice (**a**) and sagittal oblique CT slice (**b**). Painful ankle with multiple prior sprains: note the osseous activity on the spurs mirroring the tibia and talus (arrowheads) corresponding with anterior impingement and the bone uptake in the lateral tubercle of talus corresponding with chronic compression from posterior impingement (cf. posterior impingement page)

Evolution [12, 30]:
- Good evolution
- Factors of **poor prognosis: ankle cartilage lesion**

Principle of treatment [21]:
- Conservative Tx (+++): physiotherapy
- Arthroscopic surgery: resection of spurs and the synovitis

Discussion:
- Bone SPECT/CT is not indicated for examination of anterior ankle impingement. It can be useful in the event of suspicion of associated ankle osteochondral lesions.
- When assessing chronic pain of the ankle or foot, bone SPECT/CT can show typical signs of anterior impingement and guide the clinician [31].

Box 7

The diagnosis is clinical.

The treatment is non-operative.

Radiography is the key imaging technique to use.

The other means of imaging are useful if arthroscopic surgery is envisaged [12].

Anterolateral Ankle Impingement

Predisposition: NR
Medical history [12]:
- **Lateral collateral ligament sprain** (+++), at least 4 months ago

Frequency [12]:
- Represents more than 30% of ankle sprain sequelae

Mechanism [12]:
- Sequelae of a lesion to the anterior talofibular ligament or the ankle articular capsule with formation of a **residual fibrous tissue filling the anterolateral recess of the ankle** (Fig. 25)
- More rarely, impingement between an hypertrophied accessory anterior tibiofibular ligament and the talus dome

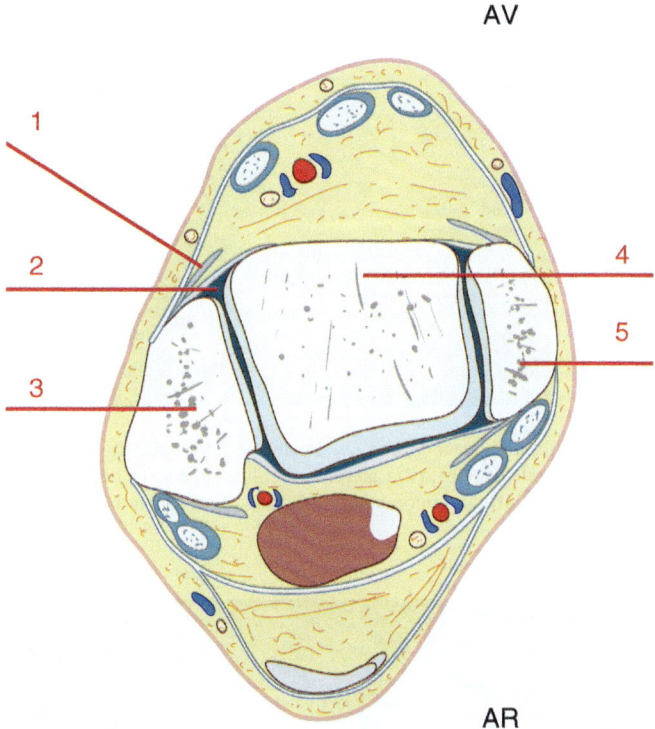

Fig. 25 Anterolateral ankle impingement, ligament and articular recess involved: transverse diagrammatic image. (1) Anterior talofibular ligament. (2) Anterolateral recess of the ankle. (3) Lateral malleolus. (4) Talus. (5) Medial malleolus

Types: NR
Interview:
- Ankle pain:
  - Chronic
  - With effort
  - Anterolateral

Clinical examination:
- Pain/pastiness upon palpation of the anterolateral gutter
- Pain with ankle flexion
- Absence of ankle instability

Paraclinical examination [12]:
- Arthro-CT/arthro-MRI:
  - Hypertrophy of the anterior talofibular ligament
  - Responsible for an irregular convexity in the anterolateral recess of the synovial cavity
- Ultrasound +/− intra-articular injection of Xylocaine in the anterolateral recess:
  - Hypertrophy of the anterior talofibular ligament
  - Injection of Xylocaine = diagnostic test and improves the visibility of the articular cavity and the impact on the anterolateral recess

Differential:
- Other causes of chronic posttraumatic ankle pain

Classification: NR
Evolution:
- Good evolution under treatment
- Factor of poor prognosis: in the event of rare associated osteochondral lesions of the talus

Principle of treatment [21]:
- Conservative Tx (++):
  - To propose to all patients
  - Physiotherapy +/− intra-articular corticoid infiltrations
- Arthroscopic surgery:
  - In the event conservative Tx fails
  - Full ablation of all altered tissues

Discussion:
- Bone SPECT/CT is not indicated for examination of anterolateral ankle impingement. It can be useful in the event of suspicion of related osteochondral lesions of the talus.

Posterior Ankle Impingement

Predisposition [12, 21]:
- **Athletes**: with movements of forced ankle extension
- Ballet dancing (+++, points), football, basketball, volleyball, etc.

Past medical history: NR
Frequency
- Dance accounts for 60% of the cases in athletes [32].

Mechanism [12]:
- **Chronic** (+++): repetitive ankle extension leads to compression of the soft tissues in the posterior region of the ankle and/or compression of the posterior process of the talus between the calcaneus and the medial malleolus [12]. Could also impact the os trigonum, whether it is fused with the lateral talus tubercle (elongated lateral process of the talus, previously "Stieda" process) or not fused (synchondrosis) [21].
- Acute: in the event of an ankle extension injury.

Types [12] (Fig. 26):
- **Bone compression syndrome:**
  - *Acute*:
    Fracture of the medial/lateral tubercle of talus
    Fracture/contusion of the os trigonum (cf. sesamoids and accessory ossicles page)
    Fracture of the synchondrosis between the os trigonum and the lateral tubercle of talus
  - *Chronic*:
    Compression of the lateral tubercle of talus (Fig. 27)
    Compression of the os trigonum
    Compression of the synchondrosis (Fig. 28)

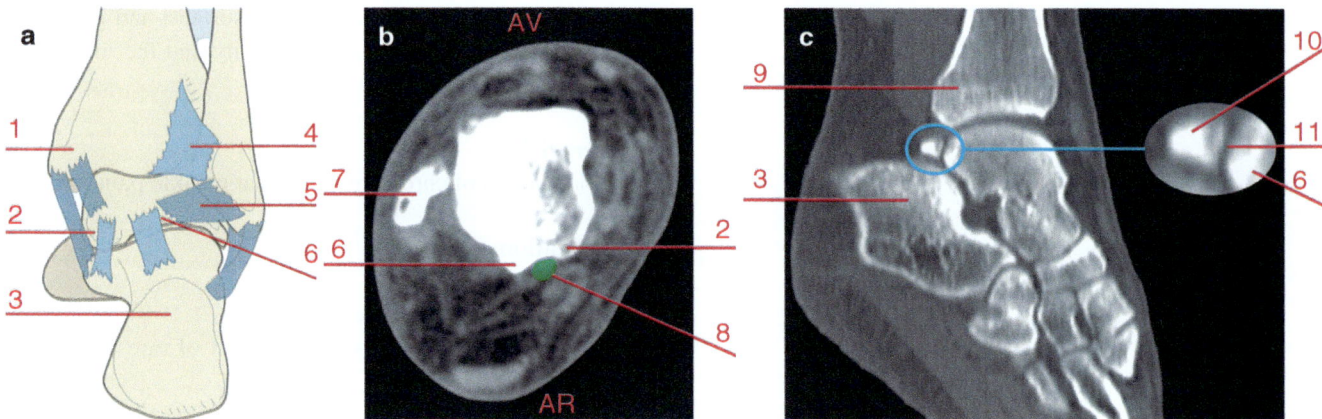

Fig. 26 (**a–c**) Posterior impingement, bone structures, and soft tissues impacted: posterior view (**a**), CT transverse (**b**), and sagittal (**c**) slices. (1) Medial malleolus. (2) Medial tubercle of talus. (3) Calcaneus. (4) Posterior tibiofibular ligament (5) Posterior talofibular ligament (6) Lateral tubercle of talus. (7) Lateral malleolus. (8) Flexor hallucis longus. (9) Tibia. (10) Os trigonum. (11) Os trigonum synchondrosis

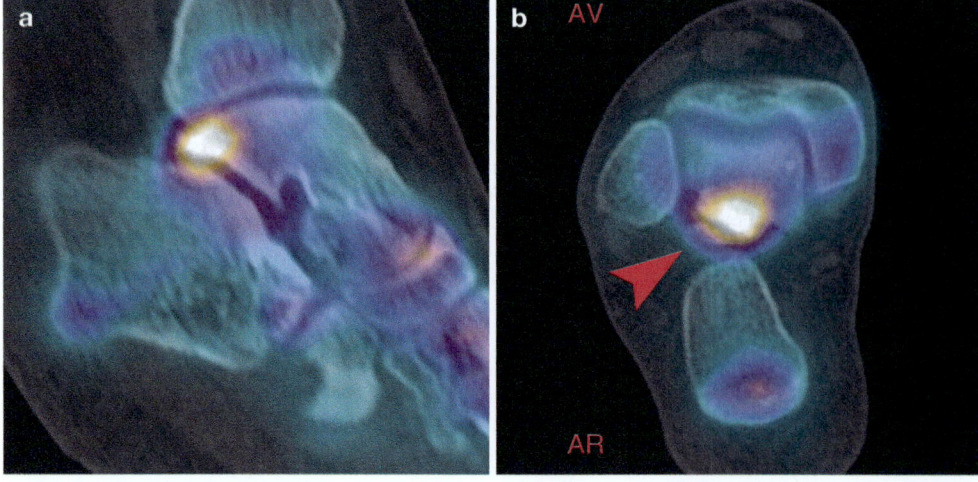

Fig. 27 (**a** and **b**) Posterior impingement, chronic bone compression of the lateral tubercle of talus: fused sagittal (**a**) and transverse (**b**) slices. Note the absence of uptake on the os trigonum (arrowhead) and synchondrosis

Fig. 28 (**a** and **b**) Posterior impingement, chronic bone compression of the synchondrosis (arrowhead), fused sagittal (**a**) and transverse CT (**b**) slices. Incidental finding in a 25-year-old asymptomatic dancer

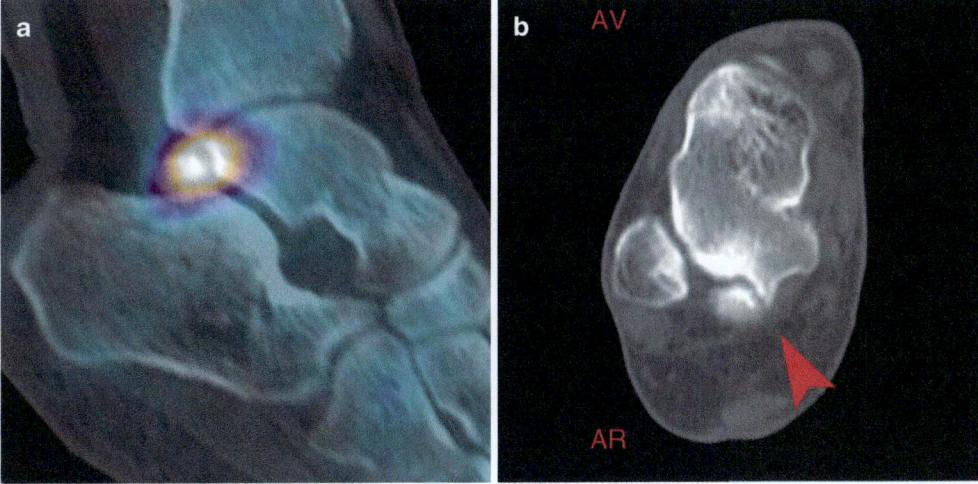

- **Soft tissue compression syndrome:**
  - *Chronic*:
    Effusion and synovitis of the ankle and subtalar articular capsules
    Tenosynovitis of the flexor hallucis longus (FHL)
    Thickening of the posterior tibiofibular, posterior talofibular, and posterior intermalleolar ligaments
- **Frequent association of bone and soft tissue compression syndrome**

Interview and clinical examination:
- Ankle pain:
  - Chronic
  - Posterior
  - Increased with ankle extension
  - With palpation of the posterior compartment

Paraclinical examination [12, 21]:
- X-ray:
  - Essential but insufficient.
  - Fractures are not very visible.
  - To see os trigonum (not very specific as often asymptomatic).
- Ultrasound:
  - To assess the articular capsule
- Bone scan:
  - To visualize bone etiology for posterior impingement (Fig. 29)
  - SPECT/CT: to specify the topography (lateral tubercle/synchondrosis/os trigonum)

- CT:
  - To examine precisely the lateral tubercle/synchondrosis/os trigonum
  - Can determine if there is a recent fracture or chronic remodeling of the synchondrosis
- **MRI** with gadolinium IV (+++):
  - To visualize the bone structure.
    Bone edema
  - To visualize soft tissues:
    Synovitis, thickening of the posterior articular capsules
    Tenosynovitis of the FHL

Differential:
- Pathology of the calcaneal tendon
- Stress fracture of the calcaneus
- Haglund disease (downward verticalization of the calcaneal tuberosity)
- OLT
- Other causes of chronic atraumatic ankle pain

Classification: NR
Evolution:
- Good evolution under treatment

Principle of treatment:
- Non-operative (+++): physiotherapy +/− infiltration
- Arthroscopic surgery:
  - In the event the non-operative Tx fails
  - Ablation of altered tissues

Fig. 29 (**a** and **b**) Symptomatic posterior impingement in an 11-year-old girl, sagittal scintigraphic (**a**) and fused (**b**) slices. Note the intense physiological activity on the growth plate of the lower tibial metaphysis (arrow), and that more moderate activity on the calcaneus tuberosity (arrowhead), not affecting the exam interpretation

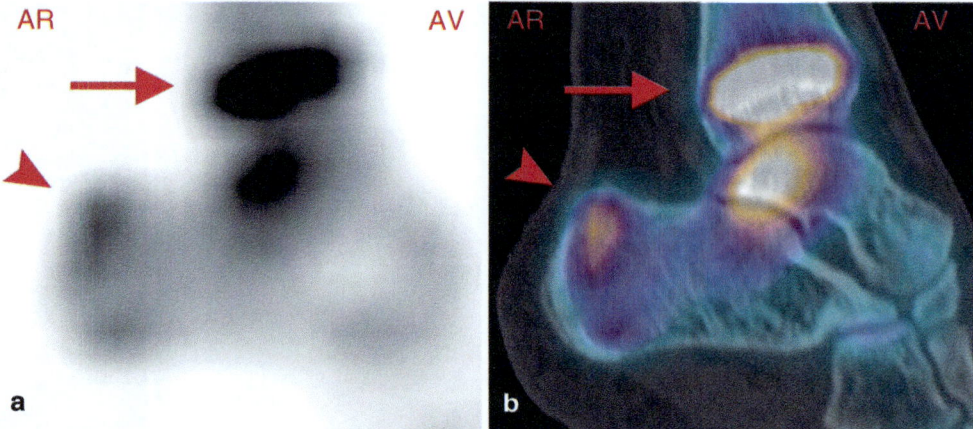

Discussion:

- The clinical assessment of impingement can be difficult, particularly in the posterior region where the involved structures are deeper than in an anterior impingement: many entities can resemble a posterior impingement [33]. When there is suspicion of impingement, standard radiography followed by MRI and ultrasound are the examinations of choice. In case of persistent doubt, a bone scan (BS) is useful for the diagnosis of posterior impingement by finding osseous etiology in the clinical symptomatology. The BS can also reveal other lesions (OLT, ankle, or subtalar osteoarthritis) [31].

- The BS can also predict surgical results: in the event of painful synchondrosis, the surgery consists of excising the os trigonum and the synchondrosis; the more uptake is anterior, overflowing onto the subtalar joint, the more the risk of post-operative residual pain increases.

Tarsal Coalition

Definition: The generic term of synostosis is poorly adapted. It is preferable to speak about tarsal coalition, which can be composed of fibrous tissue (syndesmosis or synfibrosis), cartilage (synchondrosis), or bone (synostosis) [34].

Predisposition:
- Children in their second decade (12–15 years)

Past medical history: NR
Frequency [12]:
- 1% of the general population, often asymptomatic
- Bilateral in 50% of cases

Mechanism [12]:
- Congenital.
- Abnormal bridge of tissue between two bones, present from birth.
- Ossification can be full: progressive ossification of the bridge leads to a decrease in mobility and the appearance of pain usually starting in a person's second decade.
- Ossification can be incomplete: the bridge can be made of cartilage (synchondrosis) or fibrous tissue (synfibrosis). The bridge can be well tolerated and asymptomatic, explaining the frequency of the incidental findings at adulthood.
- Can impact all foot bones (Fig. 30), but it touches the calcaneus in 90% of the cases.

Types [12, 35]:
- **Calcaneonavicular synostosis (50%)** (Fig. 31):
    - Complete: osseous bridge between the anteromedial part of the anterior process of calcaneus and the inferolateral edge of the navicular

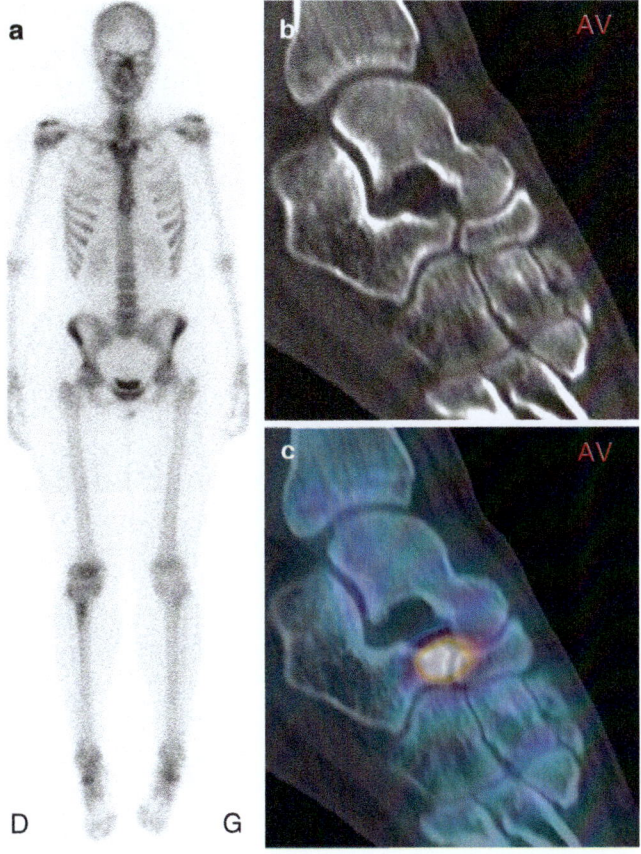

Fig. 31 (**a–c**) Bilateral calcaneonavicular synchondrosis, anterior view of WB (**a**), sagittal CT (**b**), and fused (**c**) slices. Twenty-six-year-old woman, surgical patellar translation of the right knee 7 months prior, persistence of pain: suspicion of CRPS I. Global moderate uptake in the right knee, without osteoarthritic uptake of the articular surface of the patella on the SPECT (not shown): aspect compatible with a CRPS I in the warm phase. Fortuitous discovery of a bilateral and symmetrical moderate uptake of the tarsi, which could not correspond to osteoarthritis in this young patient: a second SPECT-CT found an asymptomatic bilateral synchondrosis

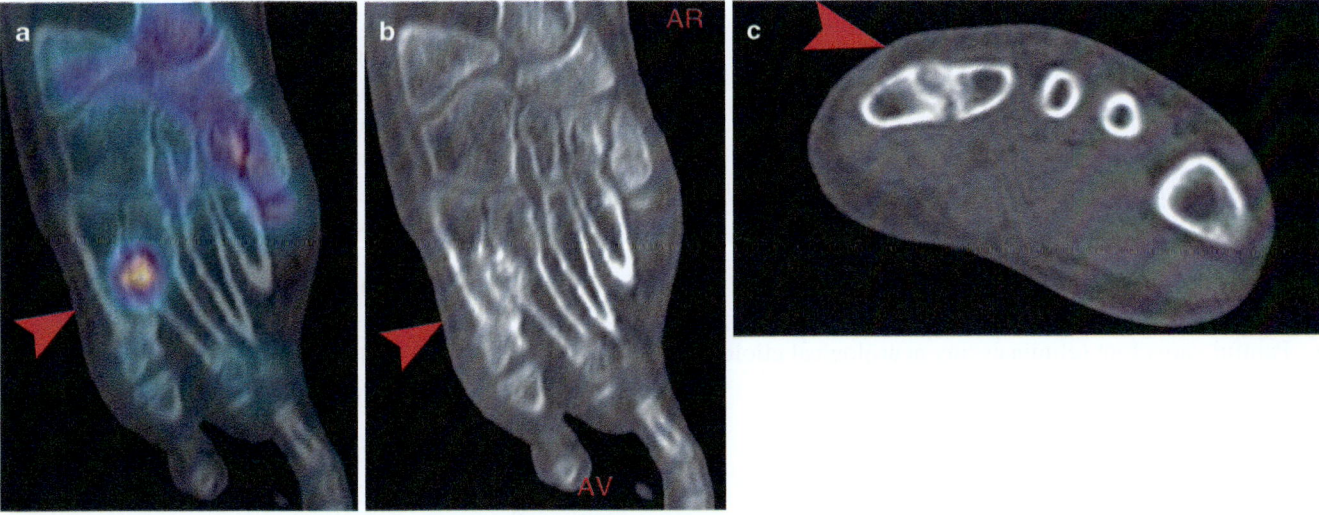

Fig. 30 (**a–c**) Recurrent M4–M5 synostosis, transverse fused (**a**) and CT (**b**) slices, coronal CT slice (**c**) of the right foot. Nine-year-old girl, operated for bilateral M4–M5 synostosis 4 and 2 years prior on the left foot and 4 years prior on the right foot: recurrent M5 pain on the right foot

Fig. 32 (**a–d**) Talocalcaneal synchondrosis, left foot, frontal CT (**a**) and fused (**b**) slices, sagittal CT (**c**) and fused (**d**) slices

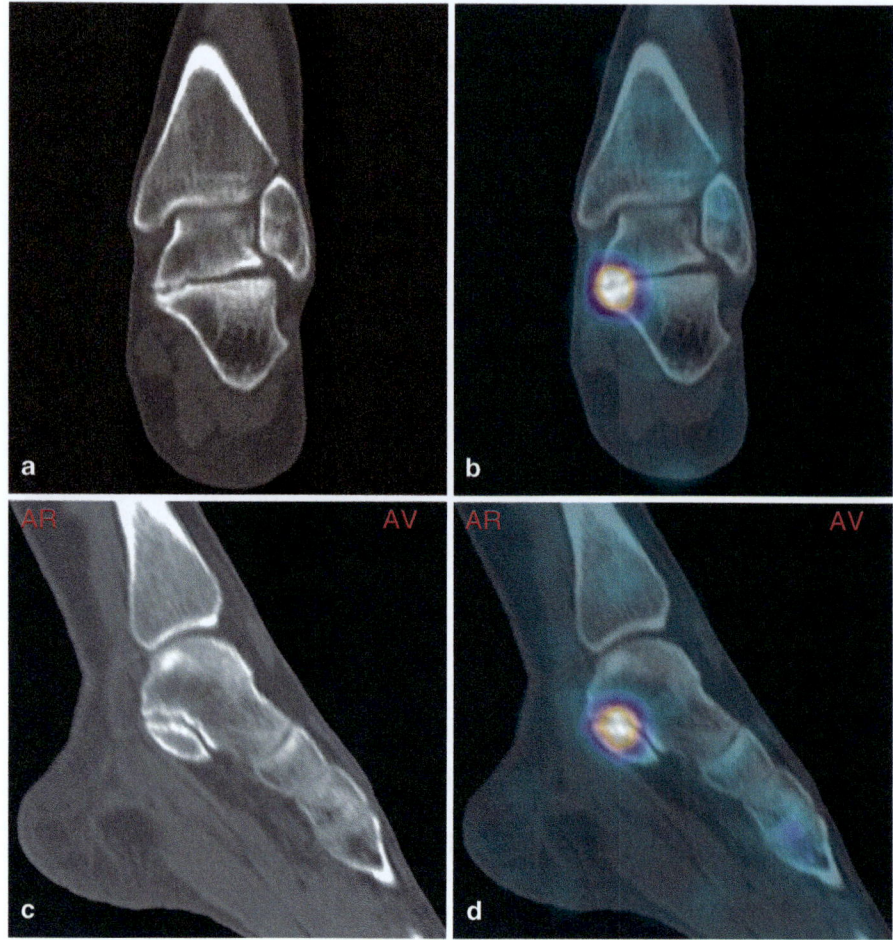

- Incomplete: resembles pseudarthrosis; lengthening of the large calcaneus process
- **Talocalcaneal synostosis (40%)** (Fig. 32):
  - Complete: medial osseous bridge, between the sustentaculum tali and the medial process of talus
  - Incomplete: resembles medial pseudarthrosis; possible talar beak (dorsal outgrowth from the head of talus by capsular traction due to a dysfunction of tarsal mobility) (Fig. 33)

Interview:
- Mechanical pain
- Repetitive sprains on rough ground (the subtalar joint can no longer adapt)

Clinical examination:
- Stiff, irreducible, and painful valgus flatfoot
- Painful varus foot (eliminate any neurological etiology)

Paraclinical examination [35]:
- X-ray (+++):
  - Often sufficient in the event of calcaneonavicular synostosis: to visualize the osseous bridge

- Difficult interpretation in the event of talocalcaneal synostosis: classic "double C" radiographic image of the calcaneus hard to discern
- CT (++):
  - In case of clinical doubt:
    To confirm or disprove the diagnosis
    To determine the exact localization of the bridge and its size
    To find other synostoses
  - In the event of synchondrosis and synfibrosis:
    To visualize the pseudarthrosis aspects with irregular and condensed banks
- Bone scan (++):
  - Essential in the event of synostosis/synchondrosis/synfibrosis:
    Confirms the zone of osseous impingement
    Must correspond to painful symptomatology
  - Can fortuitously find synchondrosis/synfibrosis that is not very symptomatic in an adult

Differential:
- Ankylosis: acquired synostosis (post-infectious, traumatic, inflammatory, etc.)

Fig. 33 (**a–c**) Talar beak and incomplete talocalcaneal synostosis, fused frontal slice (**a**), sagittal fused (**b**) and CT (**c**) slices. Fifty-five-year-old man, known left talocalcaneal synchondrosis not very symptomatic, recent pain aggravation. Note the clear uptake of the synchondrosis (arrowhead), and the more moderate uptake on the dorsal outgrowth of the head of talus (arrows), representing capsular ankle traction due to a dysfunction of tarsal mobility

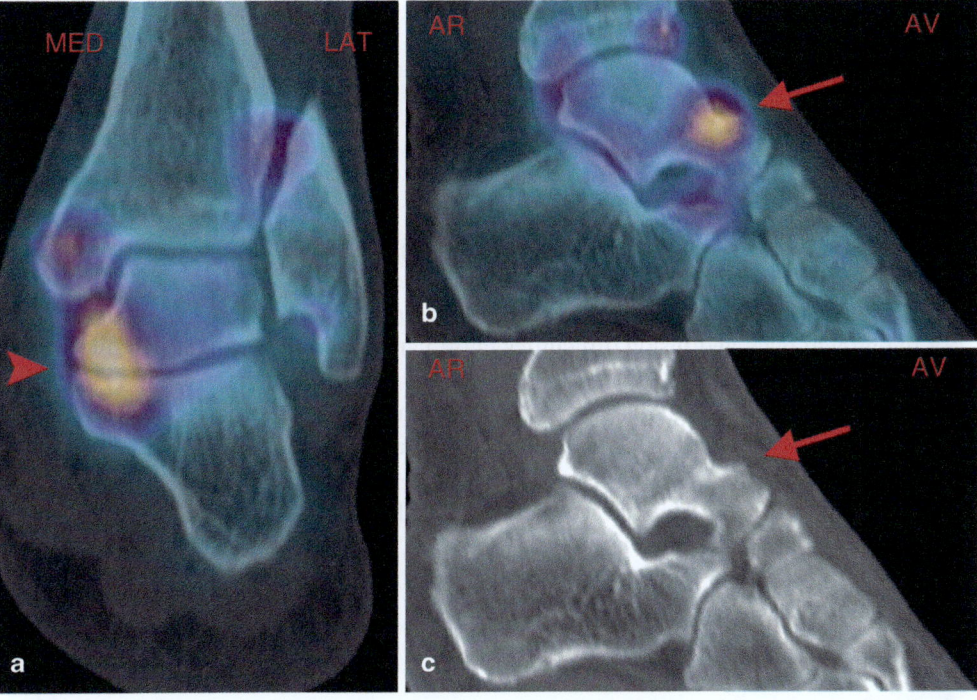

Fig. 34 (**a** and **b**) Recurrent pain after calcaneonavicular synostosis cured, sagittal fused (**a**) and CT (**b**) slices. Twenty-five-year-old man, operated for unilateral left calcaneonavicular synostosis 12 years prior, reappearance of tarsal pain a few years prior: probable insufficient ablation of synostosis

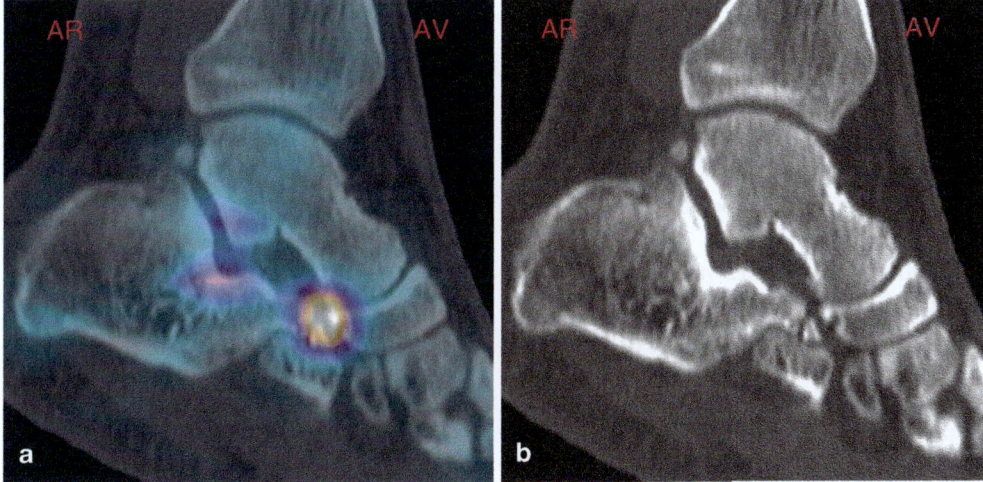

Classification: NR

Evolution:
- Irreducible deformation in valgus flatfoot

Principle of treatment [12]:
- Asymptomatic: abstention
- Not very symptomatic: rest, plantar orthotics, immobilization
- Symptomatic:
  - Single synostosis:
    Where the surface is less than one third of the articular surface: resection of the synostosis (Fig. 34).
    Otherwise: consider arthrodesis.
  - Multiple synostosis: consider double arthrodesis.

Discussion:
- A bone scan (BS) is essential for assessing synostosis in order to confirm the zone of osseous impingement. BS helps to determine the extension of a possible arthrodesis: only the zone of the synostosis or with an adjacent articulation if there is uptake.
- A BS can also prove that the synostosis is not responsible for the pain, find another cause of the patient's pains, and modify the therapeutic approach (e.g., infiltration for subtalar osteoarthritis) [36].

Box 8
Calcaneus involved in 90% of the cases

Osteochondrosis and Osteochondritis

Predisposition:
- Children and teenagers
- Often in athletes

Mechanism of the injury:
- **Osteochondrosis** (= apophysitis): lesion of an apophysis due to tendinous traction. Repeated traction by a tendon on an secondary ossification center leads to microtrauma of the growth plate and fusion difficulties in primary and secondary ossification centers [37].
- **Osteochondritis** (= epiphysitis): epiphyseal damage via mechanisms of compression and/or of metabolic origin [38]
- In both cases, the lesions touch very functionally solicited bone formations.

Types (Fig. 35):
- Osteochondrosis:
  - Calcaneal tuberosity (Sever's disease)
  - The base of the fifth metatarsal (Iselin's disease)
- Osteochondritis:
  - Navicular (Kohler-Mouchet's disease)
  - Head of the second metatarsal (Freiberg's disease, can also affect M3)
  - Lateral sesamoid (Renander's disease)

Osteochondrosis of the calcaneal tuberosity (Sever's disease) [37–39]:
- Children from 6 to 12 years
- Athletes
- By traction of the calcaneal tendon on the apophysis of the calcaneus
- Painful at the tip of the heels
- Bilateral in 50% of cases
- Impossible to walk on heels
- Paraclinical examination:
  - Not necessary if typical clinical examination and bilateral damage
  - X-ray: nonspecific densification or fragmentation of secondary ossification center
- Evolution: banal pathology, evolution without sequelae
- Principle of treatment [21]:
  - Rest from sports for several months
  - Shock-absorbing soles
  - Stretching the gastrocnemius muscles

Osteochondritis of the navicular (Kohler-Mouchet's disease) [39, 40]:
- Children from 4 to 8 years
- Limping

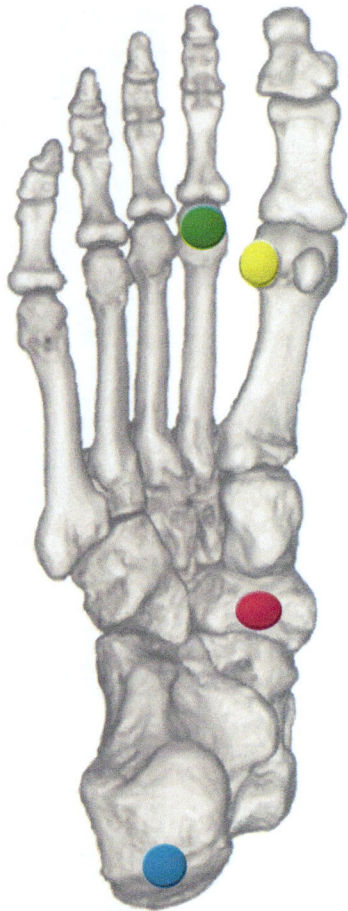

Fig. 35 Topography of the osteochondrosis and osteochondritis of the foot: plantar view. In green: osteochondritis of the head of M2 (Freiberg's disease). In yellow: osteochondritis of the lateral sesamoid (Renander's disease). In pink: osteochondritis of the navicular (Kohler-Mouchet's disease). In blue: osteochondrosis of the calcaneal tuberosity (Sever's disease)

- Pain upon palpation of the navicular
- Paraclinical examination:
  - X-ray:
    Normal at the beginning
    Then irregular/condensed/flattened navicular
  - Bone scan:
    Positive at the beginning of the disease
    Early and late hyperactivity of the navicular
- Evolution: banal pathology, evolution without sequelae
- Principle of treatment [21]:
  - Rest
  - Possible cast immobilization for 4–6 weeks
  - Support authorized depending on pain

Osteochondritis of the head of the second metatarsal (Freiberg's disease) [38–40]:
- Teenagers
- Girls

- Long second metatarsal (Greek foot)
- Microtrauma (running, combat sports, dance)
- Mechanical pain under the forefoot
- Pain upon palpation of the head of M2
- Paraclinical examination:
    - X-ray: late signs, widening, and flatness of the head of M2
    - Scan: early and late hyperactivity of the head of M2
- Evolution:
    - Favorable in less than 2 years
    - Epiphyseal deformation with possible functional disability
- Principle of treatment [21]:
    - Strict rest from sports
    - Orthopedic soles
    - If ineffective, osteotomy to shorten and raise the M2

- Athletes
- Rare pathology, primarily impacts the lateral sesamoid
- Microtrauma (athletics, dance)
- Mechanical pain when stepping
- Pain upon palpation of the head of M1
- Paraclinical examination:
    - X-ray:
      Signs can appear tardily (9–12 months).
      Flattened aspect, condensed or fragmented lateral sesamoid.
- Evolution:
    - Favorable in a few months
- Principle of treatment [21]:
    - Strict rest from sports
    - Discharge orthesis

Osteochondritis of sesamoid (Renander's disease)
[21, 39, 40]:
- Teenagers
- Girls

Hallux Valgus

Predisposition [41]:
- **Women** (M/F = 1/15)
- Family heredity (25% of the cases)
- Excessive length of the first toe (Egyptian foot)

Past medical history: NR

Frequency:
- **Frequent**
- The most frequent deformation of the forefoot

Mechanism of injury [42]:
- Where there is a predisposition (anatomy, heredity, shoes, etc.), the **hallux** is directed gradually **in valgus** and the **first metatarsal in varus**. This deformation is gradually worsened by the tension from the hallucis longus tendons: (1) extensor hallucis longus which passes the lateral edge of the first MTP, as the cord of an arc, and which accentuates angulation and (2) flexor hallucis longus, between the sesamoids, which leads to a pronation of the hallux. The hallux valgus progresses, as does impingement of the medial part of the head of M1 with the shoe, causing a painful bunion. The structural modifications of the first ray and the pain have effects on the lateral rays (metatarsalgia by excessive pressure, valgus of the other toes, etc.).

Types:
- Congenital hallux valgus (before 15 years)
- Common hallux valgus
- Arthrosic hallux valgus
- Others

Interview and clinical examination [10]:
- Unaesthetic **deformation** of the **first ray**:
  - Phalanx valgus >12°
  - Metatarsal varus >10°
- Bunion:
  - Medial part of the head of M1 (Fig. 36)
  - Painful when putting shoes on

Paraclinical examination [42]:
- **X-rays** (+++):
  - Front, profile, and incidence of the sesamoids.
  - In particular, one should quantify the hallux valgus and the metatarsus varus.
  - Evaluates the anomalies in bone length of the first ray and other rays.

Differential: NR

Classification: NR

Evolution:
- Without treatment:
  - First ray: aggravation of the hallux valgus
  - Lateral rays: transfer overload (metatarsalgia, etc.), deformations

Principle of treatment [41]:
- Orthopedic:
  - Shoe recommendations
  - Relaxation orthesis
- Surgical (+++):
  - As early as possible in order to avoid the lesions of the lateral rays
  - Adapted to the size of the hallux valgus, to the patient's anatomy (short or long M1, short or long P1), and to the associated lesions
  - **Relaxation**:
    Osteotomy of the first metatarsal (scarf, chevron, etc.) And/or osteotomy of the first phalanx
  - Tx of the related lesions:
    Osteoarthritis of the first MTP: arthrodesis
    Hypermobility of the medial tarsometatarsal joint: arthrodesis (Lapidus)
    Excess length of the other metatarsals: shortening osteotomy (Weil)

Discussion:
- Bone scan (BS) does not help in the initial diagnostic assessment of hallux valgus. BS can be useful in the event of clinical suspicion of osteoarthritis associated with the first MTP without notable radiological anomalies.
- In the event of unexplained postoperative pain, a bone scan can look for complex regional pain syndrome type I, pseudarthrosis, or stress fracture.

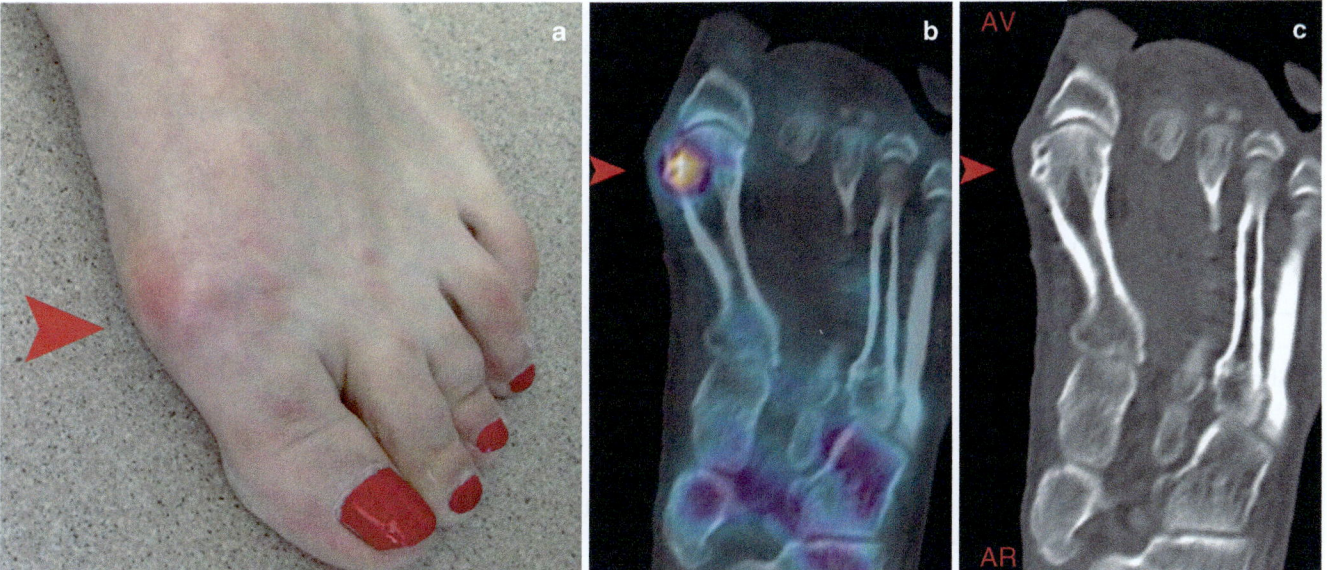

Fig. 36 (**a–c**) Hallux valgus, impingement between the medial part of the head of M1 and the shoe: photograph of left foot, anterior view (**a**), transverse fused (**b**) and CT (**c**) slices. Forty-one-year-old woman sent for pelvic pain, without SPECT-CT anomalies (images not shown). A focal uptake of the first left MTP led to a second SPECT-CT of this patient presenting a bilateral hallux valgus for 20 years, causing hindrance on the left side: uptake focused on small dystrophic lesions of the medial part of the head of M1, in connection with the bunion (arrowheads). No osteoarthritis of the first MTP, no uptake anomaly of the sesamoids

Metatarsalgia

Definition: Pain mainly located in relation to one or several metatarsal heads.

Predisposition:
- **Anomalies in the architecture of the foot**:
  - Insufficient first ray (**hallux valgus** +++, hallux rigidus, etc.)
  - Hollow foot
  - Accentuated length of the medial metatarsals
- Short gastrocnemius muscles

Past medical history: NR
Frequency: NR
Mechanism [41]:
- On a normal foot, only the heads of the first and fifth metatarsals press on the ground (cf. arch of the foot page). Metatarsalgias result from **abnormal pressure** on the heads of M2, M3, M4, or increased pressure on the heads of M1 and M5. This excessive pressure can result from (1) an insufficiency of the first ray, frequently (hallux valgus +++, hallux rigidus, etc.) (an antalgic approach aims at relieving the first ray, transferring pressure to the lateral rays); (2) A cavus foot, by excess of pressure on the metatarsal pallet; (3) A valgus flatfoot (the collapse of the medial longitudinal arch involves a calcaneal valgus and increased pressure on the first ray) (Fig. 37); (4) Accentuated length of the medial metatarsals, leading to contact of the heads with the ground; and (5) Short gastrocnemius muscles, source of ankle extension and thus of increased pressure on the forefoot.

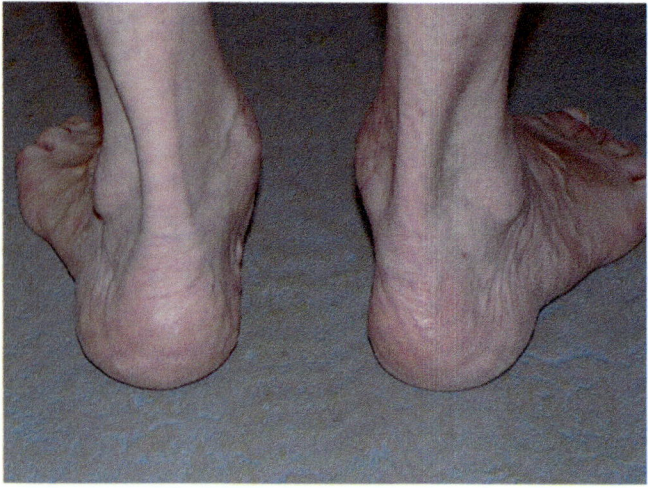

Fig. 37 Bilateral valgus flatfoot, posterior view

Types: NR
Interview and clinical examination [10]:
- Presence of an anomaly in the architecture of the foot seen in the clinical examination and with a podoscope
- Pain upon the palpation of the head of one or more metatarsals
- Hyperkeratosis under the head of one or more metatarsals (plantar callus)

Paraclinical examination [41]:
- **X-ray** (+++) (essential):
  - To evaluate the morphology of the foot
  - To eliminate certain differential diagnoses: Osteoarthritis, sequelae of Freiberg's disease (cf. osteochondritis page), sequelae of fracture
- Ultrasound (++):
  - To evaluate the plantar plate
  - To eliminate certain differential diagnoses: Morton's neuroma, bursitis, stress fracture
- Bone scan (second intention):
  - To eliminate a stress fracture or osteoarthritis
- MRI (second intention):
  - In the search of Morton's neuroma, an inflammatory pathology, etc.
- CT/arthro-CT: not very useful

Differential [41]:
- Morton's neuroma (differential diagnosis but can be associated)
- Metatarsal stress fracture
- Sequelae of Freiberg's disease
- Sequelae of fracture/contusion of a metatarsal head
- Bursitis
- Painful plantar wart (to be differentiated from pressure-related hyperkeratosis)
- Inflammatory rheumatism (RA and psoriatic rheumatism)

Classification: NR
Evolution [10]:
- Without Tx: aggravation of pain

Principle of treatment [41]:
- Adapted to the cause
- **Orthopedic** (+++): to obtain a better distribution of the pressures
  - Stretching the gastrocnemius muscles
  - Keratosis removal
  - Plantar orthesis (++), shoe recommendations
- Surgical (+++):
  - After 6 months failure of orthopedic Tx
  - **Weil osteotomy** (+++, osteotomy of metatarsal head, set with wire)
  - Tx of hallux valgus if present

Discussion:

- A bone scan (BS) is not useful in the initial assessment of metatarsalgia. However, a BS is useful for secondary elimination of a stress fracture or to look for an arthropathy; it is possible to visualize directly the overload in pressure via moderate uptake of the metatarsal head, but this is not very sensitive due to the small size of the structure and the difficulty of a perfect setting of the toes during the examination: fusion of SPECT and CT can be delicate [43]. In case of doubt about a movement artifact on the scan, it can be useful to supplement the examination with a static plantar image.
- A bone scan can have a postoperative interest, in the event of persistent pain after a Weil osteotomy.

> **Box 9**
>
> Clinical examination and radiographies are enough to diagnose the majority to the metatarsalgias.

> **Box 10**
>
> Metatarsophalangeal joint instability of the second toe (aka second crossover toe) [21, 44] (Fig. 38):
>
> - Mechanical arthropathy of the second MTP
> - With overload (can cause stress fracture)
> - Tear then rupture of the plantar plate
> - Instability, subluxation and then luxation of the second MTP
> - Favored by:
>   - First ray insufficiency (hallux valgus, short first metatarsal, etc.)
>   - Excessive length of the second metatarsal
> - Ultrasound (+++):
>   - Plantar plate: thickening, partial or complete tear
>   - +/− articular effusion/synovitis
>   - +/− bursitis under the head of M2, tenosynovitis of flexor tendons
>   - +/− stress fracture of the head of M2 or the base of P1 of the second ray

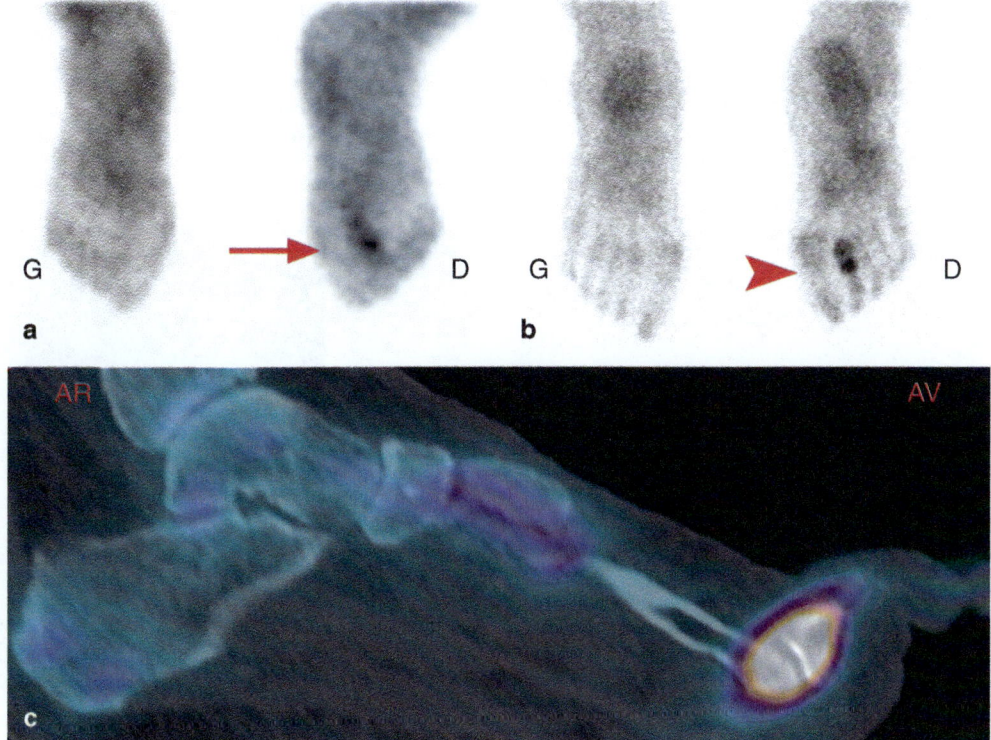

Fig. 38 (**a–c**) Metatarsophalangeal joint instability of the second toe, plantar blood pool (**a**) and delayed (**b**) images, fused sagittal slice (**c**). Seventy-seven-year-old woman, pain of the second ray of the right foot for 15 days, to eliminate a stress fracture of M2, known bilateral hallux valgus. Blood pool image shows a focal high uptake consistent with a stress fracture of the head of M2 (arrow) but SPECT-CT shows that the uptake is articular, on the second MTP. As it is difficult in these small structures to be sure that there is no movement artefact between SPECT and CT, it has been decided to supplement the examination with a static plantar image: it confirms the focal uptake is on both sides of the second MTP, predominantly on the base of P1 (arrowhead). Ultrasound performed afterward shows a slight articular effusion and a doubt on a tear of the plantar plate of the second MTP. Conclusion: metatarsophalangeal joint instability of the second toe favored by first ray insufficiency (hallux valgus), with second MTP arthropathy and probable stress fracture of the base of P1 (not seen on X-rays nor on ultrasound)

Hallux Sesamoid Disorders

General information [41]:

- They are two sesamoids, lateral and medial, under the first metatarsal head and articulated with it. They represent a point of fixation for a complex strap of ligaments and tendons **essential to effective propulsion**. A deterioration of the strap will disperse propulsion force, limiting maximal output. The hallux sesamoids receive 60% of the body weight at the end of the step and are used as shock absorbers during walking.
- We will discuss acute fractures, osteonecrosis and osteoarthritis of the hallux sesamoids. Osteochondritis (Renander's disease) and stress fractures are discussed in the corresponding chapters. The rarer disorders, such as gout, rheumatoid polyarthritis, and algodystrophy, are not discussed.

Acute fracture [21, 41, 45] (Fig. 39):

- Rare
- Medial sesamoid (+++)
- Mechanism: traumatic
  - Reception of a jump
  - Kick (martial arts)
- Sesamoid pain:
  - Brutal
  - Upon palpation
- X-ray:
  - Sesamoid fracture: irregular separation of two fragments with sharp edges
- Evolution:
  - Spontaneous: risk of osteonecrosis and pseudarthrosis (Fig. 40)
- Tx:
  - Medical (+++):
    Strapping
    Localized discharge (orthesis)
    +/− boot cast for 6 weeks
  - Surgical: if old fracture or failed medical Tx

Osteonecrosis [21, 41]:

- Rare
- Adults
- Medial and lateral sesamoids (whereas osteochondritis impacts the lateral sesamoid of athletic teenagers)
- Mechanism:
  - Vague etiology
  - Precarious vascularization
  - Can be posttraumatic or after overuse
- Pain under M1 head:
  - Mechanical, with propulsion
  - Can be inflammatory
- X-ray:
  - Flattened sesamoid
  - Irregular condensation

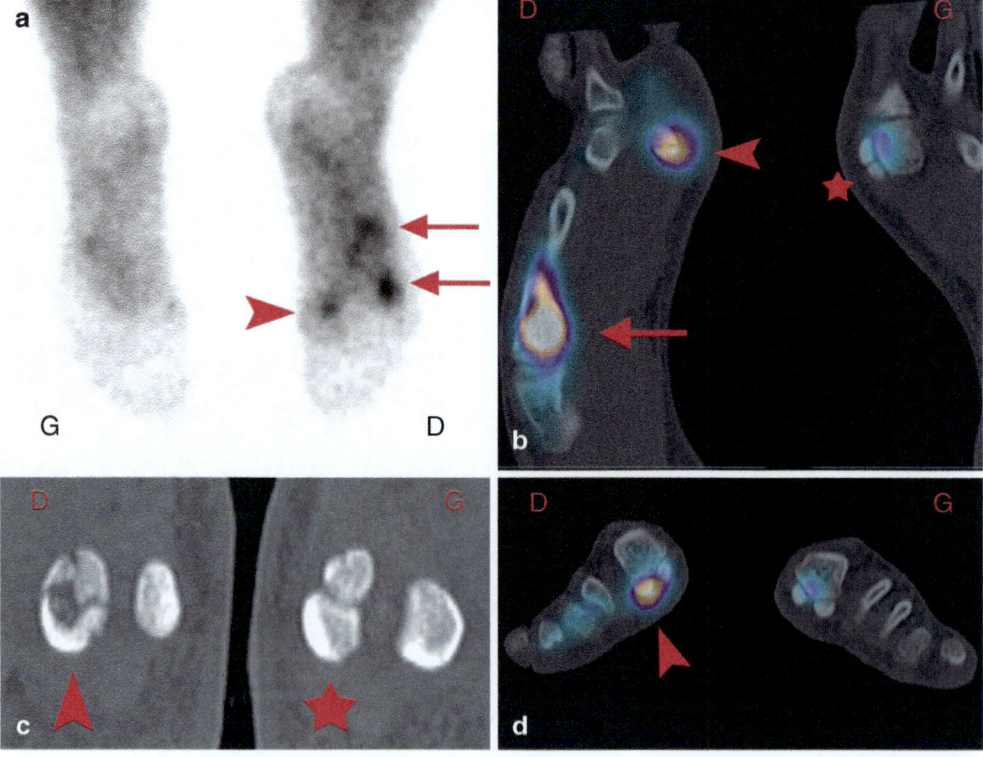

Fig. 39 (**a–d**) Acute fracture of a lateral sesamoid, plantar blood pool image (**a**), transverse fused (**b**) and thin CT (**c**) slices, fused frontal slice (**d**). Nineteen-year-old man, athlete, suspicion of stress fracture of the right M4. On the right foot, recent stress fractures of the base and head of M4 (arrows) and recent fracture of lateral sesamoid (arrowhead). On the left foot, asymptomatic bipartite medial sesamoid (star). In order to visualize the differences between fracture and bipartite sesamoids with CT, image C comes from a diagnostic thin-slice CT acquisition (which did not visualize the M4 stress fracture)

Fig. 40 (**a–c**) Sequelae of a medial sesamoid fracture, delayed plantar image (**a**), sagittal CT slice (**b**), fused frontal slice (**c**). Forty-three-year-old woman, M1 head pain and pain in the first intermetatarsal space on the left foot for the past year, without any contributing factors. Rounded uptake suggests a sesamoid disorder on the delayed plantar image, confirmed by SPECT-CT images (arrowheads). The aspect of the medial sesamoid on the CT looks more like a fracture than a split, and the absence of uptake on the plantar blood pool image (not shown) testifies to an old lesion (greater than 3 months)

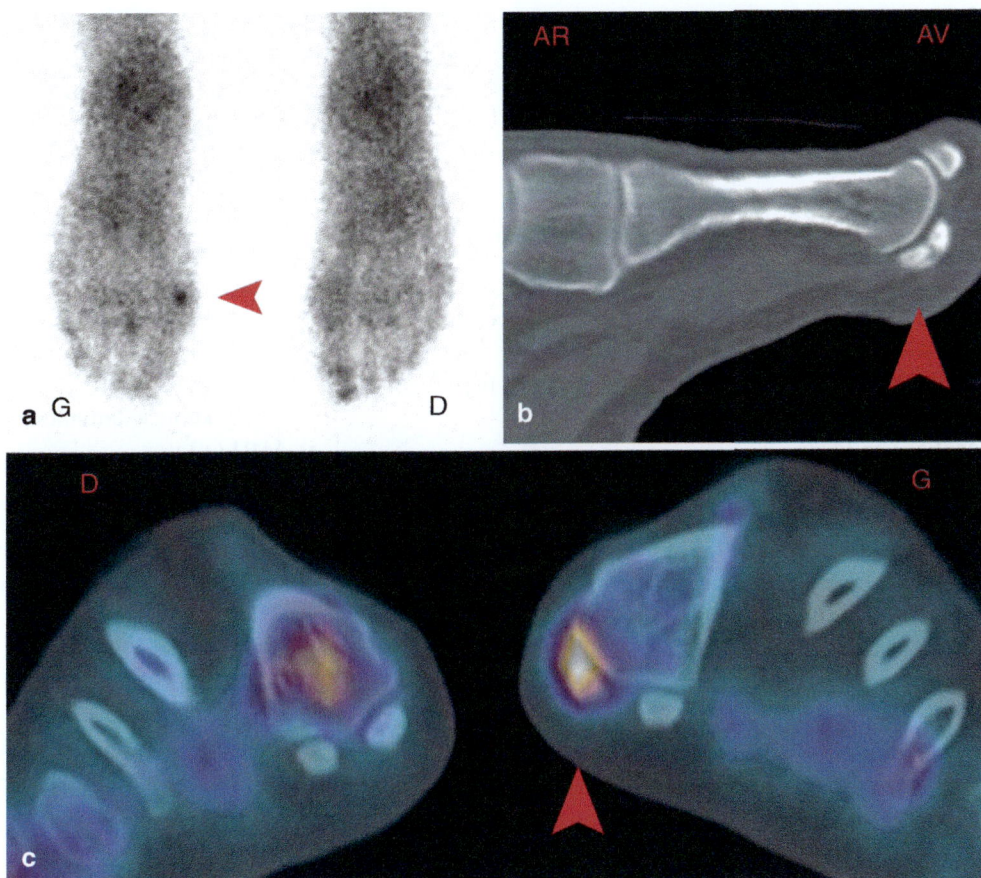

- Tx:
  - Medical (+++):
    Rest
    Localized discharge (orthesis)
  - Surgical: if medical Tx fails

Osteoarthritis [21, 41]:
- The most frequent sesamoid disorder
- Medial sesamoid (++), can touch the two sesamoids at the same time
- Osteoarthritis:
  - Primary: overuse
  - Secondary:
    Hallux valgus (+++)
    Fracture
    Hallux rigidus
- **Often well tolerated**
- Mechanical pain under M1 head
- X-ray:
  - Sesamoid: sclerosis
  - Posterior osteophyte
- Tx:
  - Medical (+++):
    Rest
    Localized discharge (orthesis)

Box 11
Medial sesamoid [41]:
- Often larger than lateral sesamoid
- More often bipartite
- More in contact with the head of M1
- **More overused and most prone to traumatic and degenerative pathologies**

Bipartite:
- Frequent (≈15% of the patients), may be bilateral
- More frequent (≈30%) in the case of hallux valgus
- Medial sesamoid (+++)
- X-ray: two rounded and regular bone fragments

Morton's Neuroma

Predisposition [41]:
- **Women** (M/F = 1/4)
- **50 years** (30–70 years)

Antecedents: NR

Frequency:
- **Frequent**
- Excessively diagnosed, precise prevalence difficult to evaluate
- Incidence ≈ 150 by 100,000 person-years [10]

Mechanism [41]:
- **Tunnel syndrome** responsible for an irritation of the interdigital nerve, generally caused by a fibrous tumefaction of this nerve (pseudoneuroma). The precise etiology is not known; several mechanisms have been suggested: (1) shearing with microtrauma to the nerve at the third intermetatarsal space, due to mobility between the talar foot (including the three first metatarsals) and the calcaneal foot (including the two last metatarsals); (2) wearing of high heels among women leading to hyperextension of MTP articulations and plantar compression of the nerve against the intermetatarsal ligament; and (3) bursae, presenting only in the second and third intermetatarsal space, which can become inflamed (bursitis), favoring local inflammation followed by fibrosis of the nerve.

Types [46]:
- Typical clinical form: most frequent
- Atypical clinical forms:
  - Night pain
  - Constant pain
  - Feeling like there is an internal foreign body

Interview [10]:
- **Plantar pain**:
  - **Mechanical** (walking, trampling, driving)
  - Progressive, then **violent**/paroxysmal
  - With sensation of burning/electric charge irradiating toward the toes
- Of the **third** (+++) or second (+) **intermetatarsal space**
- Requiring patient to stop using the foot for support, removal of shoes, and the mobilization of the forefoot

Clinical examination [41]:
- Pain caused with the transverse squeezing of the metatarsal heads together with one hand and simultaneously compressing the intermetatarsal space with two fingers of the other hand: **painful click** of the fibrous nodule (Mulder's sign, nearly pathognomonic).
- Sense neurological disorder on both sides of the intermetatarsal space, frequent.

Paraclinical examination [46]:
- Examinations can eliminate a differential diagnosis, quantify the lesion, and look for related injuries before starting a treatment.
- **X-ray:**
  - Always done.
  - Often normal; look for a differential diagnosis.
- **Ultrasound (+++):**
  - Done in a second phase
  - Very sensitive and very specific
  - Can visualize the neuroma (nodular thickening of the nerve >5 mm)
  - Dynamic examination: ultrasound Mulder's sign
- **MRI (++):**
  - Done in a third phase, in case of diagnostic doubt or before surgery.
  - To visualize the neuroma (Fig. 41)
  - To visualize related lesions/differential diagnoses:
    Bursitis
    Bone lesion
    MTP lesion

Differential [41, 46]:
- **Bursitis** (differential diagnosis or can often be associated with the neuroma)
- MTP lesion:
  - Synovitis
  - Osteoarthritis
  - Second crossover toe (lesion of the plantar plate under the MTP, with dorsal subluxation of the toe on M2, cf. metatarsalgia page)
- Bone lesion:
  - **Stress fracture**
  - Osteochondritis of the M2 head (Freiberg's disease)
- **Metatarsalgia** (differential diagnosis or can often be associated with the neuroma)

Classification: NR

Evolution [46]:
- Spontaneous evolution: chronicity
- Better results if dealt with fast

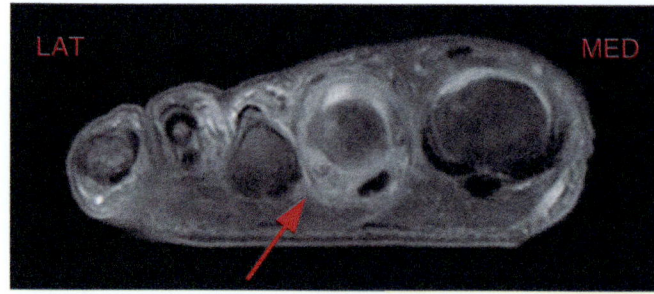

Fig. 41 Morton's neuroma, frontal MRI view, T1 fat sat gadolinium. Thickening of the interdigital nerve of the second space (arrow)

- **Under medical Tx:**
  - Shoes and orthesis: improvement in 40% of cases
  - Local corticoid injection: improvement in 80%, transitory
  - Radiofrequency: improvement in 80%
- **If surgery:**
  - Improvement in 90% of cases
  - Possible recurrence

Treatment [41]:
- **Medical (+++):** decrease the pressure on the foot:
  - **Adapted shoes:** not too tight, no high heels
  - **Plantar orthosis.**
  - Stretching the gastrocnemius muscles
  - Local injection: corticoids/analgesics
  - Radiofrequency (thermal ablation of the neuroma)
- **Surgery:** if medical Tx fails.
  - Neurectomy: ablation of the nerve.
  - Neurolysis: freeing the nerve.
  - Postoperative care must be **nonpainful**, to avoid painful post-amputation nerve pain.

Discussion:
- Bone scans do not contribute to diagnosing Morton's neuroma.
- In case of diagnostic doubt in spite of the X-ray/ultrasound couple, the MRI is the examination of choice: The neuroma as well as the possible related bursitis or metatarsalgia can be visualized on the same coronal view. In the event of inconclusive MRI, a bone scan could possibly be done, notably to look for a stress fracture.

Box 12

Morton's neuroma is frequent and nuclear physicians must be familiar with its typical clinical form, even if bone scans are not indicated in standard assessment.

- 50-year-old women
- Pain/irradiant paroxystic burn
- Of the third (+++) or second (+) intermetatarsal space
- Occurring with pressure
- Yielding at rest and when shoes are removed

Box 13

Ultrasound and MRI can visualize a thickening of the interdigital nerve >5 mm, which does not mean that it is the cause of the pain [46].

Tendon Disease

> **Box 14**
> **Definitions** [47]:
> **Pathology of the tendon: tendinopathy**
> - Lesion of the enthesis: enthesopathy
>   - Inflammatory: enthesitis
>   - Mechanical: enthesosis
> - Lesion of the body of the tendon: corporeal tendinopathy
> - Lesion of the myotendinous junction: myotendinous tear
>
> **Pathology of the tendon's environment:**
> - Lesion of the paratenon: paratenonitis (aka peritendinitis)
> - Lesion of the synovial sheath: tenosynovitis
> - Lesion of the retinaculum or the flexor pulley

In the event of a strict tendon pathology, without bone lesions, delayed bone scan images are generally normal. In addition, because of weak resolution in contrast, the CT of SPECT-CT is not appropriate to evaluate the tendons and the synovial sheaths. By taking account of these limitations, the objective of this chapter is to present various tendon disorders and to specify the SPECT-CT signs which point to a tendinous etiology of foot or ankle pain. Bone lesions that could be related to tendon disorders are covered because they can be seen on bone scans. We will treat the tendon groups of the anterior, medial, lateral and posterior ankle [48] and plantar talalgias (Fig. 42).

Anterior Ankle Tendon Group

Tibialis anterior [15, 41]:
- Infrequent disorder.
- The most medial tendon of the anterior part of the ankle finishes on the medial edge of the first cuneiform and the medial edge of the base of M1.

- *Corporeal tendinopathy*:
  - Not very frequent
  - Mechanism: mechanical (excessive effort, shoes too tight)
  - Older women
  - Pain/impotence:
    With flexion of the ankle while walking
    On the tendon path
    Increased with palpation

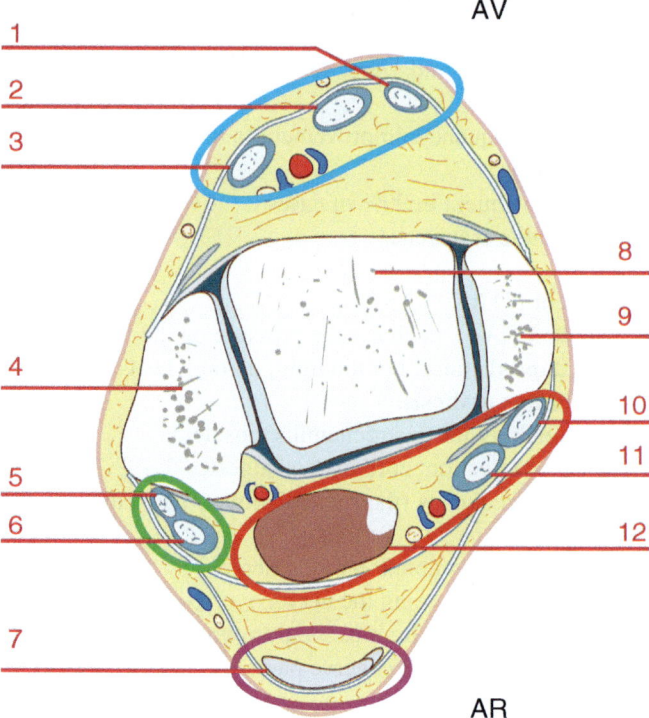

Fig. 42 Tendon groups of ankle: axial diagram cut through the ankle joint. Surrounded in blue: anterior group. Surrounded in green: lateral group. Surrounded in red: medial group. Surrounded in purple: posterior group. (1) Tibialis anterior tendon (2) Extensor hallucis longus tendon (3) Extensor digitorum longus tendon (4) Lat. malleolus (5) Fibularis brevis tendon (6) Fibularis longus tendon (7) Calcaneal tendon (8) Talus (9) Medial malleolus (10) Tibialis posterior tendon (11) Flexor digitorum longus tendon (12) Flexor hallucis longus

- Ultrasound +/− MRI: corporeal tendinopathy
- Tx: medical (+++)
  Rest
  Analgesics +/− NSAIDs
- *Enthesopathy*:
  - Rare
- *Tenosynovitis*:
  - Not very frequent
  - Mechanism: inflammatory (rheumatoid arthritis)
  - Clinical examination: ≈ idem corporeal tendinopathy
  - Ultrasound/+/−MRI: tenosynovitis
  - Tx: medical (+++):
    Rest, immobilization
    +/− corticoid infiltration

Extensor hallucis longus and extensor digitorum longus:
- Very rare pathology

Medial Ankle Tendon Group

Tibialis posterior [12, 17, 42, 48]:
– Frequent disorder.
– The tendon is retromalleolar medial, the most anterior and medial in the group. It passes under the medial malleolus and runs forward along the medial talus surface. Approximately 2 cm before the navicular bone, it divides into two to three bundles: a main bundle fits primarily on the tuberosity of the navicular (via or not an accessory navicular). The remainder of the tendon passes under the foot and inserts into all the other bones of the tarsus (except the talus) and on the bases of M2, M3, and M4. The tibialis posterior tendon provides important support for the medial longitudinal arch of the foot: insufficiency of this tendon is one of the major causes of flatfoot.

• *Enthesopathy*:
  – Frequent
  – Mechanism:
    Degenerative (+++):
      Without accessory navicular
      With accessory navicular (++): present in approximately 15% of the patients and very often bilateral; it is classified into three types, and type II is generally symptomatic (Figs. 43 and 44).
    Traumatic: tear of navicular tuberosity (Table 1).
  – Ultrasound: enthesopathy
  – MRI (+++): enthesopathy
    +/− edema of the tuberosity of navicular.
    If accessory navicular: look for fracture or necrosis, and evaluate the synchondrosis.

– Bone scan (++): intense medial tuberosity uptake
– Tx:
    Medical (+++):
      Rest, immobilization
      Orthesis
    Surgery:
      Accessory navicular:
        In the event of failure of medical Tx
        Excision of the accessory bone and repair of the tendon

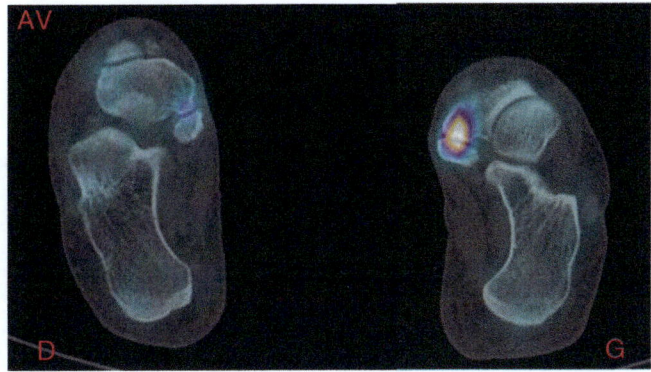

Fig. 44 Bilateral accessory navicular type II, intense uptake on the left: transverse CT slice

Table 1 Difference between an accessory navicular type II and an avulsion fracture of the navicular tuberosity

	Accessory navicular type II	Avulsion fracture of the navicular tuberosity
Acute trauma	No	Yes
Bilateral	Yes (50–90%)	No
Size	9–12 mm	<10 mm
Aspect	Regular, corticalized	Irregular

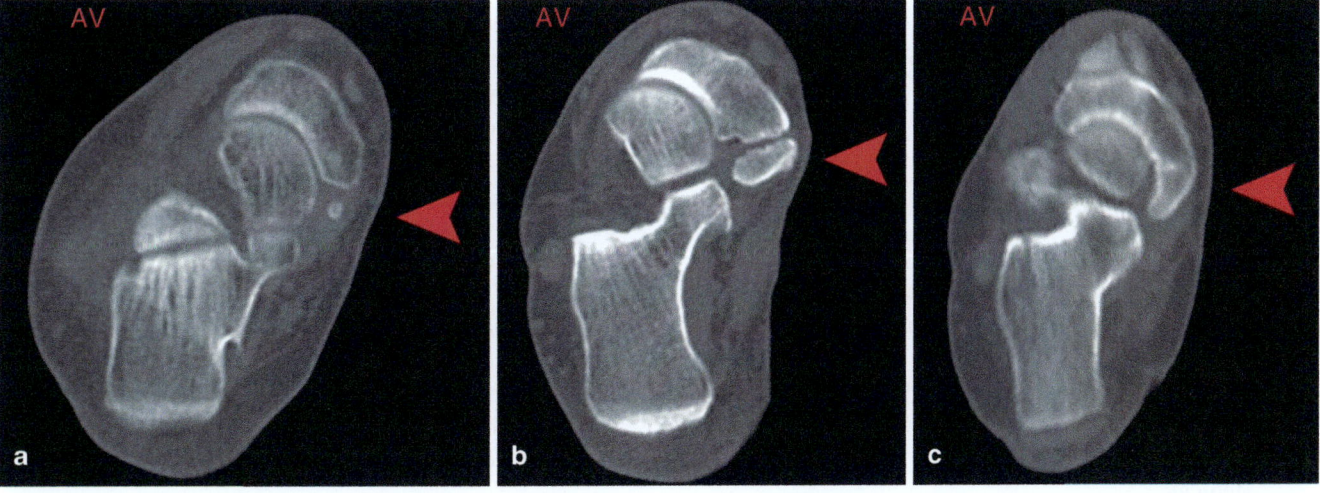

Fig. 43 (**a–c**) Accessory navicular type I (**a**), type II (**b**), and type III (**c**): transverse CT slices

Fig. 45 (**a–d**) Corporeal tendinopathy of the tibialis posterior, front view of blood pool phase (**a**), transverse fused (**b**) and CT (**c**) slices, fused sagittal slice (**d**). Thirty-year-old man, examination of left foot pain for the past 8 months. Note the linear medial uptake on the blood pool phase (arrowhead). The osseous uptake on image **b** translates the impingement between the posterior cortical of the medial malleolus and the thickened tendon: visible tendinous thickening on the image **c** (arrow). Note also on the same foot (image **d**), a plantar fasciitis and an enthesopathy of the quadratus plantae (confirmed by MRI); the calcaneal enthesopathy is not evolutive

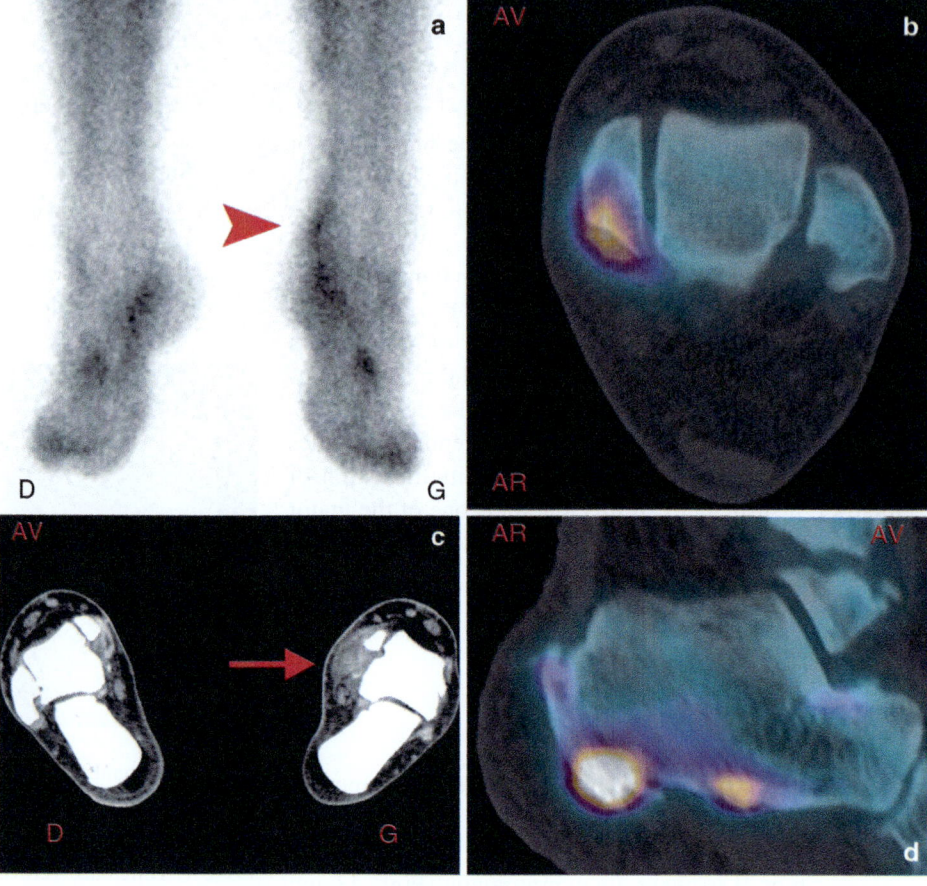

Tuberosity tear:

    Recent: strict immobilization or surgery

    Old: based on clinical tolerance

- *Corporeal tendinopathy* (Fig. 45):
  - Frequent
  - Mechanism:

    Degenerative (+++)

    Athletic overuse (abrupt changes of direction: basketball, tennis, etc.)
  - Women, > 50 years, overweight
  - Pain behind/under medial malleolus or medial longitudinal arc
  - Flatness of the foot, unilateral
  - X-ray: flatness of the foot
  - Ultrasound/MRI:

    Corporal tendinopathy.

    +/− tenosynovitis.

    Look for lesions of the plantar calcaneonavicular ligament (spring ligament), frequently related to this injury.

    +/− osseous edema of the medial malleolus (bone and tendon conflict, visible on MRI).
  - Tx:

    Medical:

        Rest

        Orthesis

Surgery:

    Tendon suture

    +/− Relaxation of the back of the foot

- *Tenosynovitis* (Fig. 46):
  - ≈ idem corporeal tendinopathy
  - Mechanism: can be inflammatory (RA)
  - Tx:

    Medical (++):

        Rest, immobilization

        +/− corticoid infiltration

    Surgery:

        Synovectomy

        +/− relaxation of the back of the foot

Box 15

The presence of an accessory navicular weakens the insertion of the tibialis posterior tendon.

In the event of an accessory navicular of type II, the tibialis posterior tendon fits directly onto the additional bone, without plantar insertion, resulting in overconstraint on the tendon and synchondrosis, followed by weakening of the medial longitudinal arch [42].

Fig. 46 (**a** and **b**) Tenosynovitis or corporeal tendinopathy of the tibialis posterior, post-fracture of P1 of the fifth toe: blood pool phase (**a**) and delayed image (**b**), anterior view. Sixty-nine-year-old man, direct impact on the fifth left toe 6 weeks prior, debilitating pain and normal radiographies. For the past 4 weeks, pain and tumefaction on the medial part of the left ankle. Note the linear medial activity, more intense on blood pool than on delayed image, testifying to a tendinous pathology (arrow) and the recent fracture of P1 of the fifth toe (arrowhead)

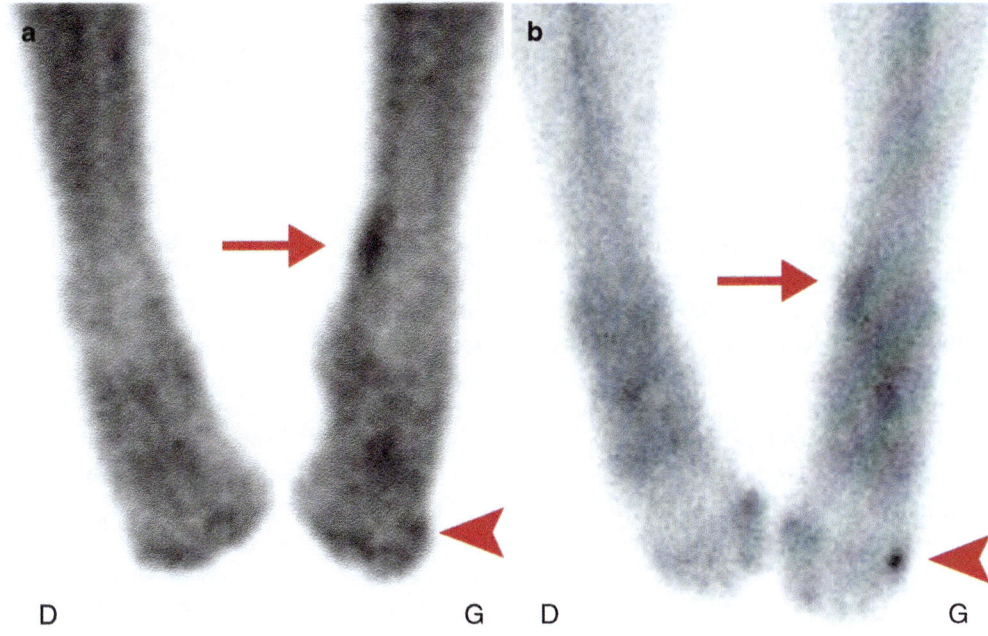

Flexor hallucis longus [41]:

– The body of the muscle runs down rather low to reach the ankle, and then the tendon passes in the groove between the lateral and medial tubercles of the talus. It passes under the medial part of ankle and then under the sustentaculum tali and fits into the base of P2 of the hallux.

• *Corporeal tendinopathy*:
  – Not very frequent
  – Mechanism:
    Overuse (sports requiring a strong impulse on the fore-foot: dance, running)
    Posterior impingement (cf. posterior impingement chapter):
      Lesion of the posterior process of the talus
      Osteophyte of subtalar osteoarthritis
      Muscle body abnormally low in conflict with the groove between the lateral and medial tubercles of the talus
  – Pain/impotence:
    When standing on the tip of the toes
    Medial retromalleolar and retrotalar
    Increased upon palpation and the opposing flexion of the hallux
  – Ultrasound +/– MRI:
    Corporeal tendinopathy.
    Look for posterior impingement.
  – Tx:
    Medical (+++):
      Rest, immobilization

• *Tenosynovitis*:
  – ≈ idem corporeal tendinopathy
  – Mechanism: can be inflammatory
• *Enthesopathy*:
  – Very rare

Flexor digitorum longus:
– Rare pathology

Lateral Ankle Tendon Group

Fibularis brevis [12, 15, 21, 41, 47]:
– The tendon is in contact with the posterior edge and then goes under the lateral malleolus, running forward along the lateral side of the calcaneus and embedding at the base of M5. Behind and in the lower part of the lateral malleolus, it is maintained by the superior fibular retinaculum, which embeds into the posterolateral part of the lateral malleolus and on the lateral side of the calcaneus.

• *Corporeal tendinopathy*:
  – +/– frequent
  – Mechanism:
    Acute in the high-level athletes
    Chronic if lateral instability of the ankle: lesion to the calcaneofibular ligament with change of weight bearing to the superior fibular retinaculum and conflict of the fibularis brevis with the lateral malleolus
    Old or recent trauma, frequent

- Lateral retromalleolar pain
- Ultrasound +/− MRI: corporeal tendinopathy
- Tx: medical (++): rest + NSAIDs
- *Enthesopathy*:
  - Rare

Fibularis longus [12, 15, 21, 41, 42, 47]:
- The tendon runs behind the fibularis brevis tendon and the lateral malleolus. It passes under the lateral malleolus and runs along the lateral side of the calcaneus until it reaches the cuboid, where it changes directions, running along the groove on the plantar surface of cuboid and embedding at the base of M1. At the level of the cuboid groove, the tendon is protected by a fibrocartilaginous thickening that can ossify (os peroneum). The painful os peroneum syndrome (POPS) can represent a tendinopathy of the fibularis longus or a bone impingement with the tuberosity of cuboid (Fig. 47).

- *Corporeal tendinopathy*:
  - Rare
  - Mechanism:
    Impingement with the lateral side of the calcaneus or at the entry of the cuboid groove
    Old or recent trauma, frequent
  - Pain between the lateral malleolus and the cuboid
  - Ultrasound +/− MRI:
    Corporeal tendinopathy
    +/− fracture of the os peroneum
  - Tx: medical (++): rest + NSAIDS
- *Enthesopathy*:
  - Very rare

Fibularis longus and fibularis brevis [12, 15, 21, 41, 47]:
- *Tenosynovitis of the tendons of the fibularis longus and fibularis brevis*:
  - Synovial sheath shared by the two tendons
  - Mechanism:

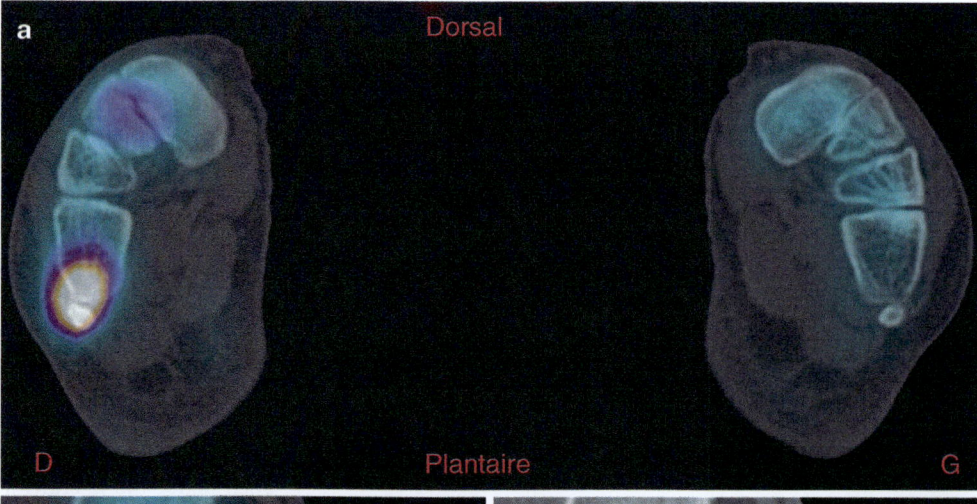

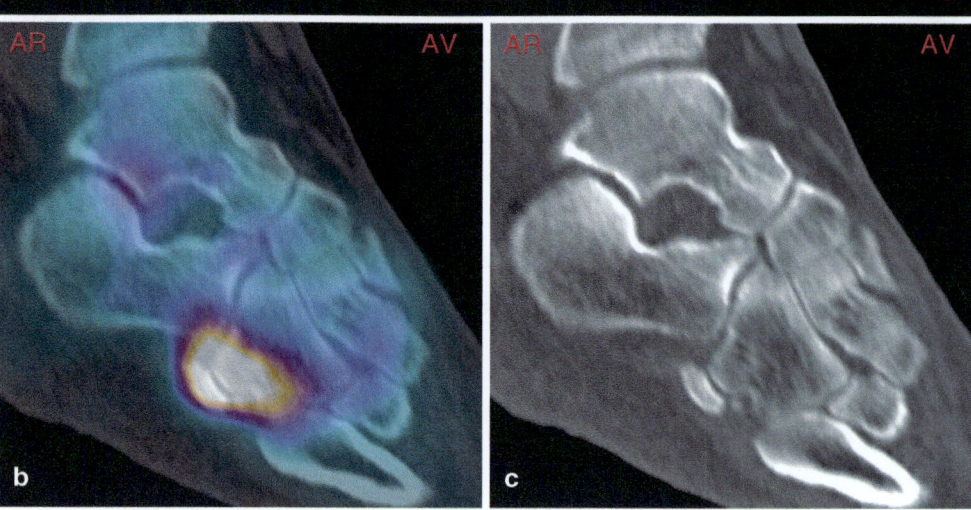

Fig. 47 (**a–c**) Painful os peroneum syndrome, fused frontal slice (**a**), sagittal fused (**b**) and CT (**c**) slices. Sixty-six-year-old woman, former athlete, lateral mechanical pain in the anterior right tarsus, evolving over the past 3 weeks, following short walking effort (1 h). Antecedents of direct impact to the lateral part of the right foot 3 months prior (fell off a stool). Note the bilateral os peroneum, symptomatic on the right: impingement between the os peroneum and the cuboid tuberosity

Posttraumatic (ankle sprain, fracture of the lateral malleolus)

Inflammatory (rheumatoid arthritis)
- Lateral retromalleolar pain
- Ultrasound/+/−MRI: tenosynovitis
- Tx: medical (+++):
Rest, immobilization
+/− corticoid infiltration

- *Dislocation of the tendons of the fibularis longus and fibularis brevis*:
  - +/− frequent
  - Lesion of the superior fibular retinaculum with or without posterior bone tears of the lateral malleolus
  - Mechanism: violent
  Trauma (ski ++)
  Forceful contraction of the peroneus muscles
  - Lateral retromalleolar pain
  - Tendinous dislocation generally spontaneously reduced and nonpalpable
  - X-ray: +/− posterior lateral malleolus tear
  - Ultrasound +/− MRI:
  Lesion of the superior retinaculum
  +/− fractures: talus, distal tibial epiphysis due to violent mechanism
  - Tx: surgical

Posterior Ankle Tendon Group

Calcaneal tendon [15, 21, 41]:
- Tears and corporeal tendinopathies of the calcaneal tendon are frequent but do not have any visualization in bone scans and will not be covered here. The calcaneal tendon has no synovial sheath, so there is no tenosynovitis in a

strict sense: inflammation of the pre- and retrotendinous synovial bursae is possible.

- *Enthesopathy* (Fig. 48):
  - Very frequent
  - Mechanism:
  Degenerative (+++), often associated with a corporeal tendinopathy
  Inflammatory: enthesitis (pso. arthritis), pre-tendinous erosive bursitis (RA, pso. arthritis)
  - 40 year of age, athletes and nonathletes
  - Posterior talalgia
  - X-ray:
  Ossification of the enthesis frequent
  +/− intratendinous calcification
  - Ultrasound/MRI: done if medical Tx fails
  Enthesopathy
  +/− Corporeal tendinopathy
  +/− Pre- or retrotendinous bursitis
  + Spongy edema of the calcaneal tuberosity
  - Tx: medical (+++)
  Rest
  Adapted shoes, heelpieces.
  +/− NSAIDS
  Caution: corticoid infiltration contraindicated because damaging
  Rehabilitation: stretching of the gastrocnemius muscles
- *Haglund syndrome*:
  - Not very frequent
  - Mechanism:
  Bony enlargement of the posterodorsal edge of the calcaneus, involving an impingement between the end of the calcaneal tendon and the shoe

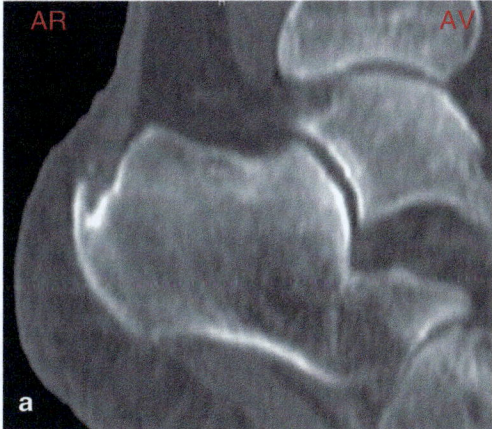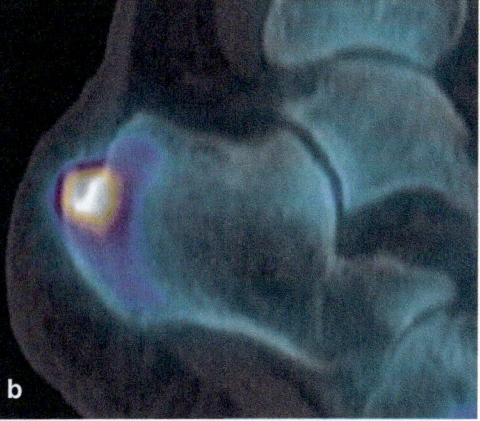

Fig. 48 (**a** and **b**) Calcaneal enthesopathy, sagittal CT (**a**) and fused (**b**) slices

Often associated with a verticalization of the calcaneus, which increases the relative posterodorsal enlargement
- Young women
- Posterior talalgia
- Irritation/cutaneous tumefaction in view of osseous overflow (impingement with shoe)
- X-ray:
  Enlargement of the posterodorsal angle of the calcaneus
  + verticalization of the calcaneus: angle >25° on image, standing profile
- MRI:
  Pre- and retrotendinous bursitis
  + spongy edema of the calcaneal tuberosity
- Tx:
  Medical: adapted shoes, heelpiece
  Surgical: if medical Tx fails
    Resection of the posterodorsal part of the calcaneus
    Osteotomy of the calcaneus
    Others: tendon plasty

Plantar Talalgia

Plantar aponeurosis [41]:
- *Plantar fasciitis (enthesopathy)* (Fig. 49):
  - Very frequent, ≈ 10% of patients during their life
  - Most frequent cause of plantar talalgia
  - Mechanism:
    Degenerative (+++), by overuse
    Excess weight, weight-bearing profession, flatfoot

- Pain:
  Of the heel when pressed
  Can decrease with walking and reappear at the end of the day
  With palpation of the calcaneal tuberosity
- X-ray:
  +/− plantar calcaneal spur, neither sensitive nor specific
- Ultrasound: proximal plantar aponevropathy (= thickening >5 mm)
- +/− MRI in the event of failure of medical Tx:
  Thickening aponeurosis.
  Spur localization: on plantar aponeurosis, flexor digitorum brevis, etc.
  + spongy edema of the calcaneus
- Differential:
  Corporeal plantar aponevropathy, more distal than plantar fasciitis
  Inflammatory rheumatism
  Stress fracture of the calcaneus
- Tx: medical (+++), during 6 weeks
  Reduction of physical activity
  Heelpiece +/− orthesis
  Stretching plantar aponeurosis and gastrocnemius muscles
- Evolution:
  Possible spontaneous resolution
  Under medical Tx: resolution >80% of cases

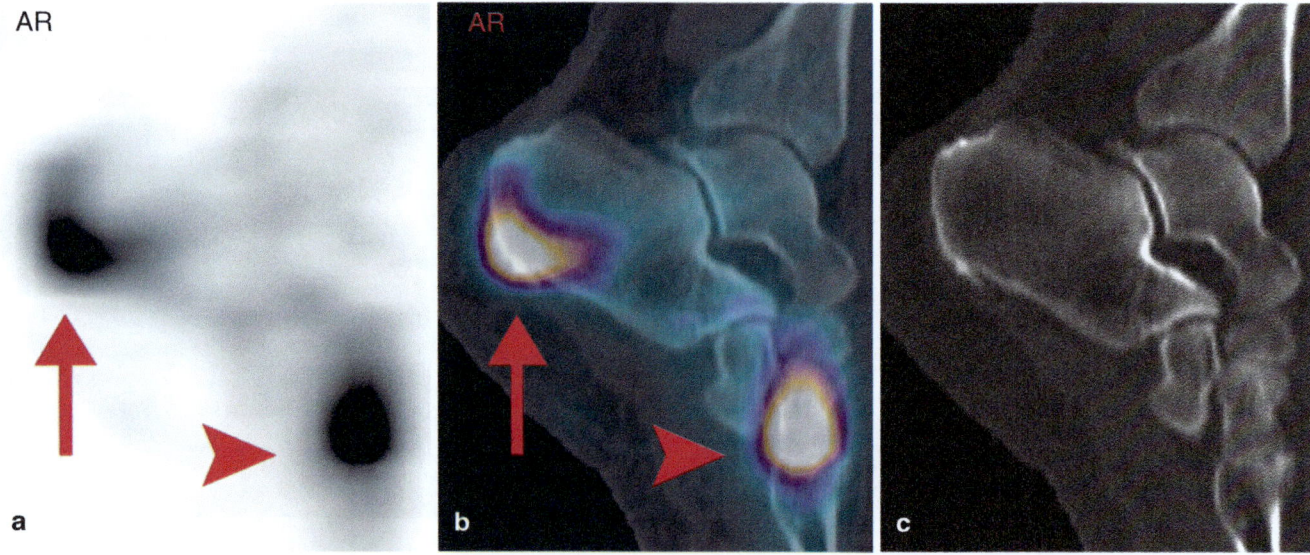

Fig. 49 (**a–c**) Recalcitrant right plantar fasciitis, increased pain over 6 weeks: intense uptake of the known enthesopathy (arrow) and finding of recent stress fracture of lateral cuneiform (arrowhead). Sagittal SPECT (**a**), fused (**b**) and CT (**c**) slices

Box 16

Corporeal tendinopathy and tenosynovitis: signs on ultrasound and MRI

- Corporeal tendinopathy:
  - Ultrasound:
    Thickened tendon, hypoechogenic, fuzzy edges
    Synovial sheath: +/− light effusion
  - MRI:
    Thickened tendon, T1 hyposignal, moderate heterogeneous T2 hypersignal
    Synovial sheath: +/− light effusion in T2 fat sat hypersignal

- Tenosynovitis:
  - Ultrasound:
    Tendon +/− heterogeneous
    Synovial sheath: clear effusion
  - MRI:
    Tendon +/− heterogeneous
    Synovial sheath: clear effusion in T2 fat sat hypersignal

NB: With MRI, the normal tendon is in T1 hyposignal and T2 hyposignal.

Box 17

Corporeal tendinopathy and tenosynovitis: signs on bone SPECT-CT

- Blood pool phase:
  - Intense linear uptake drawing the tendon/synovial sheath
- Delayed phase:
  - Could be normal
  - +/− very moderate cortical uptake translating the osseous impingement with the thickened tendon
  - +/− thickening/calcification of the tendon/synovial sheath (CT window analysis of soft part)

A bone SPECT does not allow to distinguish between corporeal tendinopathy and tenosynovitis. The distinction must be made using ultrasound or MRI.

Bone Tumors of the Ankle and Foot

This chapter does not set out to describe all bone tumors of the foot and ankle, but to focus on the most frequent, which can be discovered using bone SPECT-CT and for which CT imagery is characteristic: Only the osteoid osteoma and the simple bone cyst will be described. Bone tumors of the foot and ankle are rare (≈3% of skeletal tumors) and are primarily benign (>80% of the cases) (Table 2) [9, 21].

Osteoid Osteoma [21, 41] (Fig. 50):

- Most frequent, ≈20% of foot bone tumors
- Highly vascularized benign tumor, classically intracortical: On the foot, osteoid osteomas can be intraspongious, subperiosteal, or articular. It is composed of a small lacunar round zone of 10 mm maximum (nidus), very often including central sclerosis. It is evolutionary, causing intense peritumoral edema.
- Children, adults, **young people** (M > F)
- Foot pain:
  - **Inflammatory** (even permanently)
  - Relief with **aspirin** (+++, on the foot, this sign can be absent in the event of related synovitis.)
- CT: looks like a **target**
  - Gap ≤10 mm (nidus, can be absent)
  - Central sclerosis (can be absent)
  - Peripheral sclerosis
- Bone scan (++):
  - Early and delayed intense focal uptake
- Topography: impacts the talus (neck +++) > calcaneus (near talocalcaneonavicular joint) > rest of the foot
- Tx: if typical, no biopsy
  - Percutaneous radiofrequency ablation (+++ on foot localizations)
  - Surgery (Tx of choice if surgical access easy)
- Evolution under Tx:
  - Immediate disappearance of pain

Simple bone cyst [21, 41] (Fig. 51):

- ≈5% of foot tumors
- Asymptomatic, fortuitous discovery
- CT:
  - Pure osteolytic lesion
  - Ballooned, regular
  - Filled of liquid
  - Thin peripheral sclerosis
- Bone scan:
  - No early or delayed uptake
- Impacts the calcaneus (+++, 1/3 anterior)
- Tx: none, exceptional pathological fracture

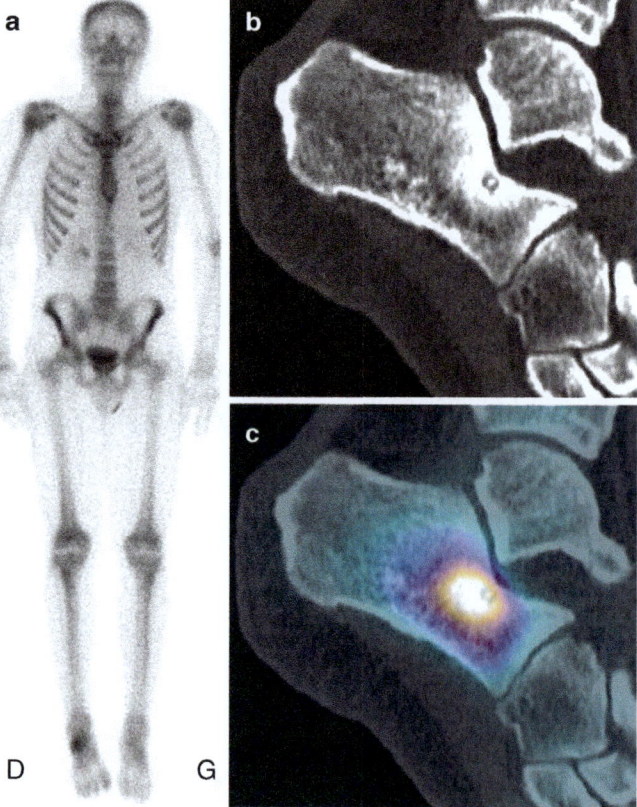

Fig. 50 (**a–c**) Osteoid osteoma of the right calcaneus: anterior view of WB (**a**), sagittal CT (**b**), and fused (**c**) slices. Twenty-two-year-old man, handball player, pain in the right foot. The initial bone scan (BS, not shown), carried out without SPECT-CT, showed an intense uptake in the calcaneus, suggestive of a stress fracture. Persistence of pain 1 year later, calcaneal edema on MRI: a new BS shows intensive uptake in the right foot on the WB view (**a**), corresponding to an osteoid osteoma under the calcaneal periosteum on CT (**b**) and SPECT-CT (**c**) slices. This case illustrates the need for obtaining SPECT-CT images when performing BS of the foot. Note the typical target lesion on the image B (Images from Dr. P. Cambefort)

Table 2 The most frequent bone tumors of the foot

Histology	Frequency (%)
Osteoid osteoma	≈20
Enchondroma	10–15
Osteochondroma	5–10
Simple bone cyst	5–8
Aneurysmal cyst	5–7
Chondroblastoma	4–8

All these histologies are benign

Fig. 51 (**a** and **b**) Simple bone cyst of the calcaneus, sagittal CT (**a**) and fused (**b**) slices. Typical CT image, no uptake, fortuitous discovery

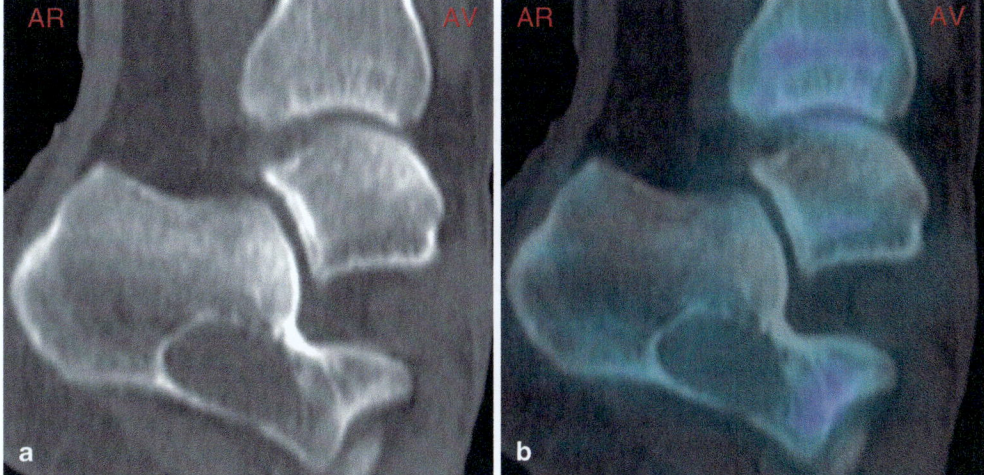

Pseudarthrosis (Nonunion)

Definition:

- "Pathological entity characterized by ossification failure following a fracture, with the inability to form normal callus, leading to the existence of a 'false joint' (thus the name) [49]."
- *Pseudarthrosis*: absence of consolidation of a fracture after 6 months
- *Delayed union*: absence of consolidation of a fracture between 3 and 6 months

Predisposition, past medical history, and risk factors [50]:

- Linked to trauma:
  - Open fracture (unpreserved perifractural hematoma)
  - Major bone loss
  - Severity of soft injury
  - Infection
- Linked to fracture site:
  - Local constraints (Fig. 52)
  - Terminal vascularization
  - Prior radiotherapy
- Linked to the patient:
  - Smoking (++, due to vasoconstriction and hypoxia)
  - Advanced age
  - Osteoporosis
  - Diabetes mellitus
  - Medications: NSAIDs (++, alters inflammatory phase of bone callus), corticoids
- Linked to healthcare:
  - Missed fracture (Fig. 53)
  - Poor contention
  - Non-conservation of the perifractural hematoma (in the event of plate osteosynthesis) (Fig. 54)
  - Lesion of the periosteum (in the event of plate)
  - Persistence of an interfragmentary space (in the event of intramedullary nail)

Frequency:

- ≈10% of fractures are complicated by nonunion or delayed union.

Mechanism:

- After a fracture, **normal bone healing** occurs by callus, in **four stages**: (1) **Inflammatory stage** (from D0 to D4): formation of a hematoma, rich in inflammatory cells (monocytes/macrophages, platelets, etc.) secreting local growth factors allowing the recruitment and differentiation of osteoprogenitor cells for the bone marrow, the cortical bone, and periosteum. (2) **Soft callus formation stage** (from D4 to D28): the hematoma is invaded by fibroblasts, chondroblasts, and osteoblasts that will produce a very vascularized fibrocartilaginous matrix which gradually will replace the hematoma. (3) **Hard callus formation stage** (from D28, for 2–3 months): the cartilaginous matrix is replaced by an osseous matrix. (4) **Bone remodeling** (from the third month, prolonged several months): the hard callus is transformed into normal corticalized bone [50, 51].

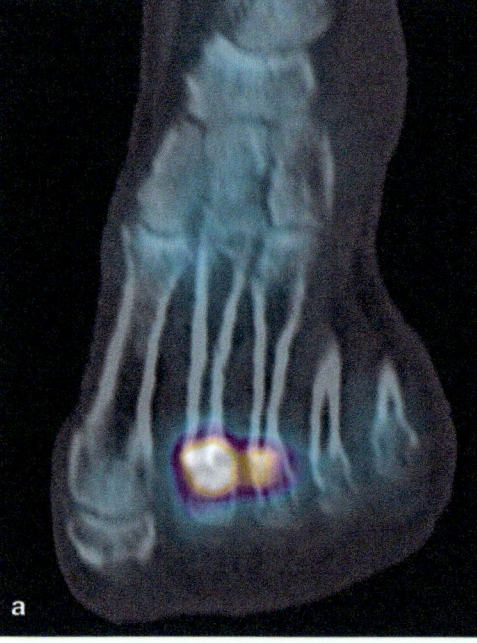 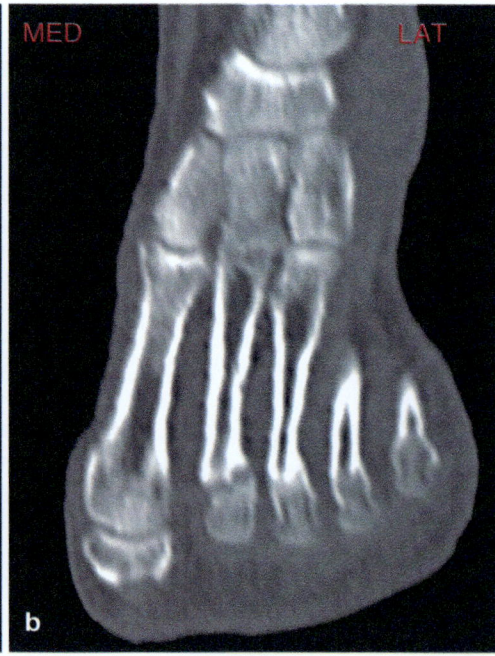

Fig. 52 Pseudarthrosis on osteotomy, transverse fused (**a**) and CT (**b**) slices. Thirty-nine-year-old woman, osteotomy of the necks of M2, M3, M4, and M5, 22 months prior for round foot. Persistence of pain: pseudarthrosis of the neck of M2 and the neck of M3 to a lesser degree. Good consolidation of M4 and M5

Fig. 53 (**a** and **b**) Atrophic pseudarthrosis of the medial malleolus, frontal CT (**a**) and fused (**b**) slices. Fifty-year-old man, car accident 3 years prior with two operated fractures of the upper limbs. Pain in left ankle since the accident, neglected and accentuating. Medial malleolus fracture, without significant uptake: atrophic pseudarthrosis on untreated fracture (arrowhead). Note the related anterolateral OLT, very evolutive (arrow)

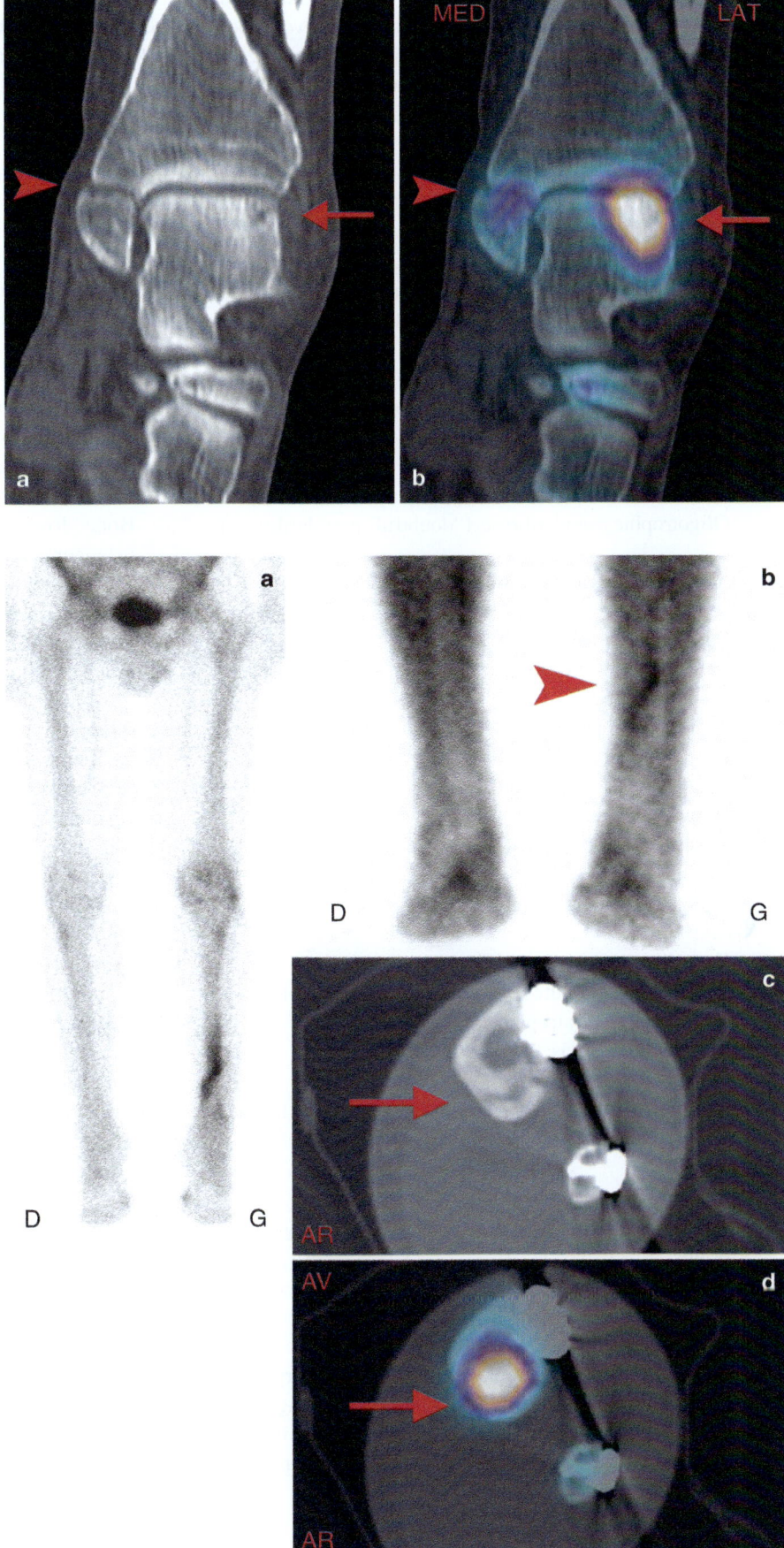

Fig. 54 (**a–d**) Hypertrophic pseudarthrosis on screw-plate osteosynthesis, front views of WB (**a**) and blood pool phase (**b**), transverse CT (**c**), and fused (**d**) slices. Fifty-seven-year-old man, left tibia and fibula screw-plate osteosynthesis 15 month prior for complex fracture, persistence of pain: CRPS I? Intense uptake on blood pool designating the fracture site, abnormal 3 months after injury and surgery (arrowhead), and intense uptake on delayed images projecting a persistent fracture line of the tibia (arrow): hypertrophic pseudarthrosis, not CRPS I

- Some micro-movements of the fracture site are tolerated because they promote callus development; however, poor contention causing abnormal mobility or shearing micro-movements (which destroy the neovascularization) will lead to pseudarthrosis. Adapted compressive forces promote consolidation by stimulation of the osteoblasts. Absence of compression and an interfragmentary space are pseudarthrosis risk factors, but an excess of compression will lead to too little callus, making it fragile. The absence of a hematoma (open fracture or plate osteosynthesis) and the loss of periosteum vascularization (major trauma, plate osteosynthesis) are pseudarthrosis risk factors.

Types:
- **Pseudarthrosis with abnormal radiographies**:
  - Atrophic pseudarthrosis
  - Hypertrophic pseudarthrosis
- **Pseudarthrosis with normal radiographies**:
  - Oligotrophic pseudarthrosis ("doubtful" pseudarthrosis)

Interview and clinical examination:
- In typical cases:
  - **Pain** with pressure
  - Persistent mobility of the fracture site
- In the doubtful cases:
  - No systematic pain
  - No obvious mobility

Paraclinical examination:
- Lab tests: WBC count, ESR, and CRP
  - Normal.
  - if ↗, suspect septic pseudarthrosis.
- **X-ray**:
  - Easy diagnosis:
    Clear visible fracture line, without bridging callus
    Hypertrophic or atrophic extremities
  - Doubtful diagnosis:
    Normal-looking callus.
    The ends of the fracture are in contact and of normal morphology.
- CT:
  - In case of radiological doubt
  - Often sufficient to visualize if there is bridging callus or not
- Bone scan:
  - In case of persistent doubt after CT
  - If suspicion of septic pseudarthrosis
- Labeled leucocyte scintigraphy with complementary bone marrow scintigraphy (cf. osteoarticular infection page):
  - If suspicion of septic pseudarthrosis, with intense uptake on blood pool and delayed images on bone scan

Differential:
- **Septic pseudarthrosis**
- CRPS I (algodystrophy)

Classification: NR

Evolution:
- Pseudarthrosis cannot heal without treatment.

Treatment:
- Etiologic Tx:
  - Mobile fracture: good immobilization
  - Patient: education, stop smoking, balancing diabetes, etc.
- **Surgery (+++):**
  - Ablation of the callus (callus not ossified if atrophic pseudarthrosis, hypertrophic callus if hypertrophic pseudarthrosis)
  - Avivement (ablation of bone necrosis)
  - Bone loss often replaced: bone graft +/− pro-osteogenic factors (BMP)
  - Addition of platelet-rich plasma (PRP)
  - Stabilization
  - Bacteriological and histological samples required to look for septic etiology

Discussion:
- **Bone scans (BS) do not contribute to diagnosing hypertrophic or atrophic pseudarthrosis**, which are easily diagnosed by the clinical examination and standard radiography. If a bone scan is done, it shows:
  - Intense uptake on blood pool and delayed images in the event of hypertrophic pseudarthrosis
  - Absence of uptake on blood pool and hypo- or normo-uptake on delayed images in the event of atrophic pseudarthrosis
- **BS can be useful to examine doubtful pseudarthrosis**:
  - Uptake on blood pool and delayed images testifies to hypertrophic-like pseudarthrosis or septic pseudarthrosis.
  - The absence of uptake on blood pool and hypo- or normo-uptake on delayed images may not eliminate pseudarthrosis (atrophic-like), but could encourage the surgeon to monitor the patient; in addition, a normal BS eliminates septic etiology (negative predictive value ≥95%).
  - Moreover, whatever the results, a BS has a legal value for the surgeon: the clinical situation (surgical gesture perceived like non-optimal by the patient) and diagnostic uncertainty can make certain patients litigious.

Box 18

All pseudarthrosis must be checked for septic etiology.

Box 19

1. **Atrophic pseudarthrosis:**

   It is the most frequent presentation (75%). It results from poor vascularization of the bone (feeder vessels cut at the time of the injury, the surgical gesture or compressed by the material used for osteosynthesis) leading to necrosis. Standard radiography shows a frayed bone, in a "radish tail," or a persistent fracture line. The diagnosis is clinical and radiological.

2. **Hypertrophic pseudarthrosis:**

   It results from anarchistic osteoblastic proliferation, favored by unsuitable use of the traumatized limb (mobilization or weight bearing too early, leading to microscopic cracks of the callus in formation). Standard radiography shows hypertrophic, "elephant foot" callus. The diagnosis is clinical and radiological.

3. **Oligotrophic pseudarthrosis ("doubtful" pseudarthrosis):**

   This is the most difficult form. The patient announces residual pain at the fracture site, and standard radiographies show normal-looking bone callus. The tomodensitometry can help in certain cases by objectively showing a cortical bridge connecting the two bone fragments, eliminating the diagnosis of pseudarthrosis. For other cases, the orthopedic surgeon is confronted with two risks: (1) suspecting pseudarthrosis when there is none, involving further surgery only to find good quality callus, and (2) missing a genuine pseudarthrosis involving monitoring and prolongation of the patient's functional impotence. In addition, it should not be forgotten that all pseudarthrosis must be regarded as septic until proved otherwise. The functional information provided by a bone scan is useful for the physician.

Box 20

Bone scan (BS) and normal osseous consolidation:

- For the blood pool (tissue) phase:
  - A few hours after a fracture, local vasodilatation and a neovascularization begin causing a major increase in vascular flow. This vascular flow is at a maximum on the 15th day, then decreases, and returns on a physiological level starting from the 12th week [50]: **Hyperactivity on blood pool phase is normal until the end of the third month post-fracture, but abnormal thereafter**.
- For the delayed (osseous) images:
  - Uptake of the diphosphonates used for the BS will be on the osteoid matrix in the process of mineralization, a phenomenon that occurs several days after a fracture: **the sensitivity of detection of a recent fracture on a delayed image of BS is 80% at 24 h and 95% at 72 h. This sensitivity of detection is better in subjects under 65 years of age: 95% at 24 h and 100% at 72 h** [52, 53].
  - Bone remodeling of the hard callus in normal bone utilizes osteoclasts (repermeabilization of the medullary canal) and osteoblasts (cortical thickening) and lasts several months, even years: **activity on delayed images is constant up to 6 months after the fracture and possible up to 2 years** (90% of the fractures are not visible any more at 2 years [52]).

Osteoarticular Infections of the Foot (Excluding Diabetic Foot)

- These are serious illnesses with major functional risks: they require early treatment with antibiotics. The antibiotherapy is initially probabilistic then adapted to the germs found with blood cultures and/or deep samples (the germs found in superficial wounds are often colonizers and do not correlate with the bacteria causing the disease). The antibiotherapy must always begin quickly but always **after** bacteriological samples have been taken.
- We will discuss acute osteomyelitis, subacute osteomyelitis (Brodie abscess), chronic osteomyelitis, acute septic arthritis, and postoperative infections.

Acute Osteomyelitis [21, 54]

Predisposition:
- Children (+++, before 3 years), teenagers.
- Adults: look for risk factors (alcohol, smoking, immunodepression, arteriopathy, and peripheral neuropathy).

Past medical history:
- Children, teenagers: no particular antecedents, an injury can precede osteomyelitis.
- Adults: initial cutaneous infection.

Frequency:
- Incidence (any localization): ≈8 per 100,000/year.
- ≈15% of acute osteomyelitides in children affect the foot.

Mechanism:
- **Children**, teenagers: hematogen contamination, attacking the osseous **metaphysis** (hypervascularized zone corresponding to the growth plate) (Fig. 55)
- **Adults**: contamination secondary to contiguous focus of infection, affecting the periosteum followed by the osseous **diaphysis**
- Germs: *Staphylococcus aureus* (+++)

Interview and clinical examination:
- Acute bone pain
- Functional impotence
- Inflammatory signs:
  - Local: swelling, redness
  - +/− general: fever, shivers

Paraclinical examination:
- Lab tests:
  - ↗ ESR, ↗ CRP
  - ↗ WBC count
  - Blood culture: +/− positive
- X-ray:
  - Late signs, after 7–10 days
  - Periosteum reaction
- Ultrasound: very useful in children
- Bone scan (+): blood pool and delayed focused intense hyperactivity
- MRI (++):
  - Imaging of reference
  - Bone edema
  - Lesion of the soft parts
  - +/− abscess
- CT (+/−): can guide deep sample taking

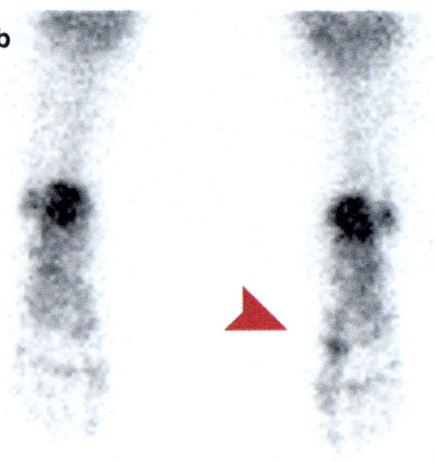

Fig. 55 (**a** and **b**) Acute osteomyelitis of M1 in a three-and-a-half-year-old girl, plantar blood pool (**a**) and delayed (**b**) images. Recent right lower limb limping: direct shock on the foot 4 days prior and fever for 24 h. Scintigraphic anomalies at the base of right M1 (arrowheads): uptake is more intense on blood pool rather than delayed images, suggesting an infection rather than a traumatic lesion. SPECT-CT imaging allows a more precise localization of the lesion (bases of M1 or tarsometatarsal joint) but is not possible without sedating the child; topography on one of the growth plate of the foot (visible on the foot contralateral and cf. pages about ossification centers of the feet) suggests acute osteomyelitis over acute septic arthritis. Clinical and biological recovery after antibiotics

Differential:
- Fracture

Evolution:
- Without Tx:
  - Aggravation: fistulization, septicemia
  - Orthopedic complications compromising the growth in children
- Blind ATB: chronic osteomyelitis
- Adapted Tx: usual recovery

Treatment:
- Medical (+++):
  - Rest
  - ATB:
    Probabilistic followed by adapted
    IV followed by PO
    4–6 weeks (4 weeks in the uncomplicated forms)
- Surgical: drainage if abscess

Subacute Osteomyelitis (Brodie Abscess) [21, 54, 55]

Predisposition:
- Children (+++, before 4 years), teenagers

Frequency:
- Incidence (any localization): ≈5 per 100,000/year.
- ≈90% of subacute osteomyelitis occurs on the femur or the tibia.

Mechanism:
- Hematogen contamination
- **Osteomyelitis circumscribed** by several factors which can be combined:
  - Increase in the host's means of defense
  - Not very virulent germ (child ≤4 years, Kingella kingae +++; children >4 years, *Staphylococcus aureus* ++)
  - Inappropriate ATB

Interview and clinical examination:
- Osteomyelitis >2 weeks
- **Rough**
- Insidious pain, of variable intensity
- Moderate functional impotence
- Inflammatory signs:
  - Local: discrete
  - General: absent

Paraclinical examination:
- Lab tests:
  - +/– ↗ ESR, often normal CRP
  - WBC count normal

- Blood culture: negative (generally not done because apyretic)
- X-ray (+++):
  - **Small lucent area within osseous sclerosis** (+++)
  - Epiphyseal, metaphyseal, or metaphysodiaphyseal
- MRI (+++), CT (+):
  - Gap filled with liquid (on the MRI, hyposignal T1 and hypersignal T2 or T2 fat sat).

Differential:
- Osteoid osteoma
- Other metaphyseal tumors or metaphysodiaphyseal tumors in children

Evolution:
- Adapted Tx: usually recovery

Treatment:
- Medical (++):
  - Rest
  - ATB:
    Probabilistic and then adapted (germ found in less than 75% of the cases, primarily by PCR assay on osseous samples)
    IV followed by PO
    6 weeks
- Surgical: to take bone samples
  - Percutaneous aspiration
  - Or drainage and curetting

Chronic Osteomyelitis [21, 56]

Mechanism:
- Complication of acute osteomyelitis
- Often favored by ATB that is not adapted

Interview and clinical examination:
- Osteomyelitis >6 weeks
- Moderate pain
- +/– moderate functional impotence
- Local and general inflammatory signs:
  - Can be absent when not in acute phase
- +/– fistula
- +/– pathological fracture

Paraclinical examination:
- Lab tests can be normal.
- X-ray (+++):
  - Cortical irregularity
  - Demineralization or lucent area, surrounded by sclerosis (Fig. 56)
  - Osseous sequestration: fragment of necrosed bone within a gap

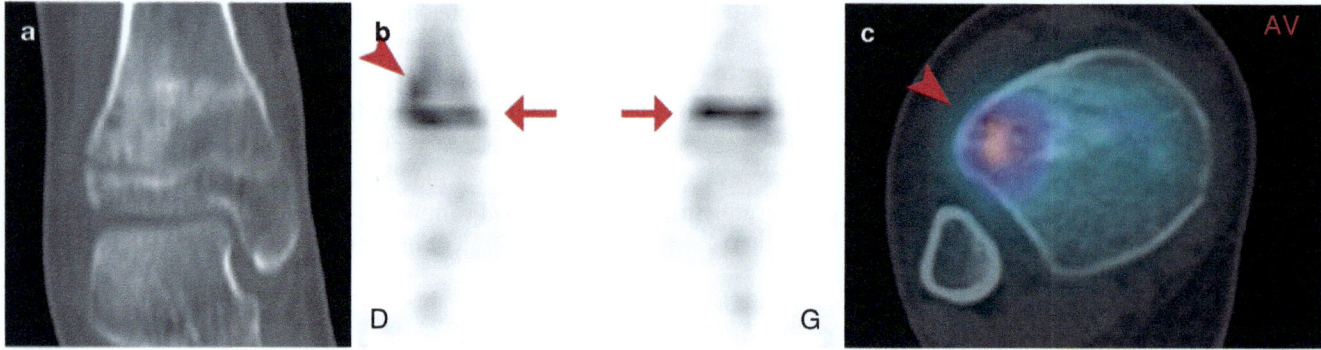

Fig. 56 (**a–c**) Chronic metaphysodiaphyseal osteomyelitis of distal extremity of the right tibia, frontal CT (**a**) and scintigraphic (**b**) slices, transverse fused slice (**c**). Twelve-year-old girl, treated for 5 months for chronic osteomyelitis, persistence of local edema and pain after 5 min of walking. Note the gaps surrounded by sclerosis and uptake testifying to the evolutive nature of the lesion (arrowhead); physiological activity of the growth plates (arrow)

- MRI (+++), CT (+/−): to assess the extent of the lesions.
- Labeled leucocyte scintigraphy (+/−): in case of diagnostic doubt.

Evolution:
- Pathology difficult to treat
- If surgical debridement insufficient: recurrence in 30% of cases
- Adapted Tx: possible cure +/− sequela
- Sequelae: pain, bone weakening, growth disturbances in children

Treatment:
- Surgical (+++):
  - Ablation of infected tissues, necrosed bone
- And medical (+++):
  - ATB:
    IV followed by PO
    6 weeks

Box 21
Inappropriate antibiotherapy:

- Blind (started **before** bacteriological samples)
- Directed against germs found in superficial samples (negative blood cultures and no deep samples taken)
- No initial IV administration, too short duration, etc.

Acute Septic Arthritis [21]

Predisposition:
- Children
- Adults

Frequency:
- ≈15% of acute septic arthritis in children affect the foot.

Mechanism of the injury:
- Hematogen contamination of the synovial fluid: quickly attacks the synovial membrane and then the cartilage and the subchondral bone
- Can affect any of the foot joints
- Germs:
  - *Staphylococcus aureus* (+++)
  - *Neisseria gonorrhoeae* (++, sexually active young adults)
  - *Streptococcus*
- Rare cases of contiguous spread and by penetrating injury

Interview and clinical examination:
- Acute pain in the articulation
- Stiffness
- Inflammatory signs:
  - Local: swelling, redness
  - General, usually present: fever, shivers

Paraclinical examination:
- Lab tests:
  - ↗ ESR, ↗ CRP (ESR is almost never asked for anymore in clinical practice for this kind of infection).
  - ↗ WBC count.
  - Blood culture: +/− positive.
- **Joint aspiration** (+++):
  - To find the germ
  - To eliminate microcrystalline arthritis
  - Is a diagnostic and therapeutic act
- X-ray (++): normal at the beginning
- Ultrasound (++): arthritis (effusion, synovial thickening, and Doppler signs)

Differential:
- Bursitis: less intense pain and stiffness
- Microcrystalline arthropathy (gout, chondrocalcinosis)
- Inflammatory arthritis (RA, psoriatic arthritis)

Evolution:
- Without early adapted Tx: articular destruction
- Under Tx: usually cured

Treatment:
- Medical (+++):
  - Rest
  - ATB:
    Probabilistic followed by adapted
    IV followed by PO
    3 weeks
- Surgical (+++):
  - Early joint aspiration and/or drainage

Post-operative Infection with Orthopedic Material [21]

- Very rare, risk increases with:
  - Complexity of the operational gesture
  - Quantity of osteosynthetic equipment
  - Patient (alcohol, tobacco, etc.)
- The MRI, which is a very good tool for the assessment of osseous infection, can be very bothered by the artifacts generated by the prosthetic metal.

Classification:
Several possible classifications [57, 58]:
- Based on postoperative delay (Zimmerli-Trampuz):
  - *Early infection* (≤3 months): clinical symptomatology is clear with local signs and fever, biological inflammatory syndrome.
  - *Delayed infection* (>3 months): torpid evolution, the patient never feeling "well" with the prosthesis/material, the clinical and paraclinical assessments are difficult.
  - *Secondary infection* (hematogenous on sepsis): rarer, begins suddenly with a prosthesis that had been fine before.
- Based on surgical management (Tsukayama and Coventry classification, which we will use):
  - *Acute infection* (≤3 weeks): possibility of simple washing without ablation of the material.
  - *Chronic infection* (>3 weeks): must change the material due to bacterial biofilm installation.
  - *Secondary infection* (hematogenous on sepsis): when caught early (less than 3 weeks before the beginning of the symptoms), it can be treated like an acute infection; if not it is treated like a chronic infection.

Type:
Superficial postoperative infection: infection of the soft tissues

- **Acute:**
  - +/− painful
  - Inflammatory signs:
    Local: swelling, redness, heat
    General: generally absent
  - No abscess, sinus tract or osseous contact
  - Tx:
    Medical (+++):
      ATB for 10 to 15 D
- **Chronic:**
  - Eliminate any deep subjacent infection (+++)
  - Otherwise, same Tx as superficial acute infection

Deep postoperative infection: osteitis, abscess, and sinus tract
- It is very difficult to make a precise diagnosis between superficial infections, deep infections, and banal postsurgical remodeling.
- Paraclinical examinations can be obstructed by the presence of osteosynthesis material.
- In the event of persistent doubt between superficial infection and deep infection, Tx should be aggressive.

- **Acute:**
  - Pain
  - Inflammatory signs:
    Local: swelling, redness, heat
    +/− general: fever, shivers
  - Lab tests:
    ↗ ESR, ↗ CRP: (not very specific post-op)
  - Ultrasound, CT, MRI: look for collection, fistulization
  - Bone scan (+/−): not specific at less than 3 weeks post-op
  - Labeled leucocyte scintigraphy (+/−)
  - Tx:
    Surgical (+++):
      Surgical debridement
      Ablation of osteosynthesis material based on how long after gesture the problem appeared (+/−3 weeks)
    Medical (+++):
      ATB, IV, ≥6 weeks
- **Chronic:**
  - Indolent presentations [21]:
    Persistent pain
    Atypical superficial infection
    Scar not closing, +/− seeping

Delay in consolidation
- Lab tests:
  ESR and CRP +/– ↗
- Ultrasound, CT, MRI (+++): look for collection, fistulization, and osteitis.
- Bone scan (++):
  Good negative predictive value
  Blood pool phase: hyperactivity more than 3 months post-op = abnormal

- Labeled leucocyte scintigraphy (+/–).
- Tx:
  Surgical (+++):
    Surgical debridement
    Mandatory removal of osteosynthesis material
  Medical (+++):
    ATB, IV, 6–12 weeks

Box 22

Postoperative infection of the soft tissues: always suspect a deeper infection if:

- No fast cure of a correctly treated acute infection.
- Chronic infection.

Box 23

- Any material orthopedic is a foreign body and creates local conditions favorable to the development of infections [57–60]: bacterial adherences to the orthopedic material, development by the bacteria of a protective microfilm (slime, **biofilm**) that allows them a prolonged survival in a quiescent mode (slow growth, responsible for delayed infections) and plays the part of a filter against antibiotics and the host's immune response. The concepts of adherence and biofilm specific to the infections on material (and infectious endocarditis) explain the need for a surgical intervention with broad debridement of infected tissues, **removal of the material** if indicated, and articular washing. The quality of the surgical removal is a major predictive factor of recovery. The surgery is always supplemented by an adapted antibiotherapy, with good diffusion in the bone and the biofilm.
- Two-stage exchange is the method of reference for the chronic infections: removal of the material, free interval for 4–6 weeks without material, followed by further surgery to insert new material.
- One-stage exchange consists of removing material and reimplanting a new material in the same operational time, with debridement and washing. Using this less morbid approach depends on pre- and per-operative conditions analyzed by the surgeon (no major reconstruction needed, clear situation and known germ).
- In the event of early infection occurring within 3 weeks of the intervention (infection known as acute) or in the event of secondary infection evolving for less than 3 weeks, it could be possible to do a simple washing—synovectomy, changing the moving parts while conserving of the remainder of the material.

Box 24

Bone scan for postoperative osteoarticular infection:

- The osteosynthesis material does not impede the imaging.
- Good negative predictive value.
- Not very specific due to surgical bone remodeling:
  Blood pool phase: possible physiological activity up to 3 months post-op
  Delayed imaging: possible physiological activity up to 1–2 years post-op

---

Box 25

Labeled leucocyte scintigraphy for osteoarticular infections:

- **Two methods:**
  - In vitro: white blood cell (WBC) labeling = method of reference:
    Expensive, requires long preparation (2.5 h), withdrawal and labeling of patient's blood, an experienced radiopharmacist, heavy material (hood with laminar flow). The use of a kit (Leukokit) simplifies the procedure but does not allow for the separation of polynuclear neutrophiles (PN) from the lymphocytes.
    No allergic risk.
    Moderate diagnostic value, SE ≥ 90 and Sp ≥ 80%
    Labeling with ^{99m}Tc or ^{111}In.
  - In vivo (e.g., Leukoscan):
    Less expensive, fast preparation (10 mn), can be done in any nuclear medicine department
    Theoretical allergic risk: fragments of murine antibodies directed against the human PN
    Moderate diagnostic value, SE ≥ 85% and Sp ≥ 75%
    Labeling with ^{99m}Tc

- Osteosynthesis material does not impede the imaging.
- Is done over 2 days.
- Must be coupled with bone marrow scintigraphy: as the labeled PN accumulate in the infectious sites as well as in hematopoietic bone marrow (normal bio-distribution of the PN), bone marrow scintigraphy with labeled sulfur colloid (^{99m}Tc-Phytacis) is essential to make sure that intense labeled PN uptake does not correspond to a bone marrow site, readily ectopic following surgery.
- If ^{111}In-WBC + ^{99m}Tc-colloid: can be done on the same day. If ^{99m}Tc-WBC or ^{99m}Tc-Leu-koscan + ^{99m}Tc-colloid: there must be an interval of 2 days between the two injections.
- Criteria of positivity of labeled leucocyte scintigraphy:
  - Focused uptake at 4 h (can be diffuse in the event of septic arthritis)
  - Greater uptake at 24 h
  - No corresponding activity on bone marrow scintigraphy

Rheumatology

Osteoarthritis

Predisposition:

- H/F ≤ 1
- Age > 45 years

Past medical history:

- NR
- +/− articular or extra-articular fracture with secondary desaxation

Frequency [61]:

- **Frequent**
- Prevalence:
  - Increases with the age
  - Depends on the articulation
  - Knee:
    At 50 years ≈ 5%
    At 70 years ≈ 12%
  - Hip:
    At 50 years ≈ 2%
    At 70 years ≈ 5%

Mechanism [61]:

- Osteoarthritis is a degenerative disease of the articulations touching the articular cartilage initially (a tissue not renewed frequently), then impacting all the articular and periarticular tissues, associating a mechanical component and an inflammatory component. Mechanical constraints involve a **degradation of the articular cartilage**, with modification of the chondrocytes and of their secretion (cf. articulation page): the cartilage loses its elastic capacities gradually and is solidified. By-products of cartilage degradation released into the synovial fluid lead to **inflammation of the synovial membrane**, with activa-

tion of macrophages, T lymphocytes, and synoviocytes. The cells secrete inflammatory mediators into the synovial liquid, which are responsible for a degradation of the cartilage with progression of **joint space narrowing**. This degradation in turn leads to synovial inflammation. The mechanical constraints are also responsible for an increased remodeling of the subchondral bone:

- Osteoid substance accumulation of the cortical bone plate with thickening (**sclerosis**) and production of **osteophytes**.
- Inflammation/edema of the spongy part of the subchondral bone.
- Modification of the osteoblasts and their secretions.
- Increase in the exchanges between the bone and the cartilage (increase in the porosity and the vascularization of the cortical bone plate and the cartilage, microfractures): mediators produced by the modified osteoblasts influence the chondrocytes and take part in the degradation of the articular cartilage. At a final stage of osteoarthritis subchondral pseudokystic radiotransparent images appear (**subchondral cyst**).

Types: NR
Interview and clinical examination [61, 62]:

- **Mechanical pain**
- Stiffness
  - Time needed to loosen up in the morning does not exceed 15 min at the beginning of the disease
  - Or after an idle period
- Articulations impacted (in descending order):
  - Knees (medial compartment, lateral facet of the anterior compartment)
  - Rachis (lumbar and cervical: zygaphophyseal and symphyseal intervertebral articulations)
  - Hip (superolateral part: the sclerosis and the geodes prevail on the acetabular side)
  - Hand: bilateral and relatively symmetrical involvement of the DIP (+++, second, third, and fifth ray), of

© Springer International Publishing AG, part of Springer Nature 2018
G. Chuto et al., *Bone SPECT/CT of Ankle and Foot*, https://doi.org/10.1007/978-3-319-90811-3_2

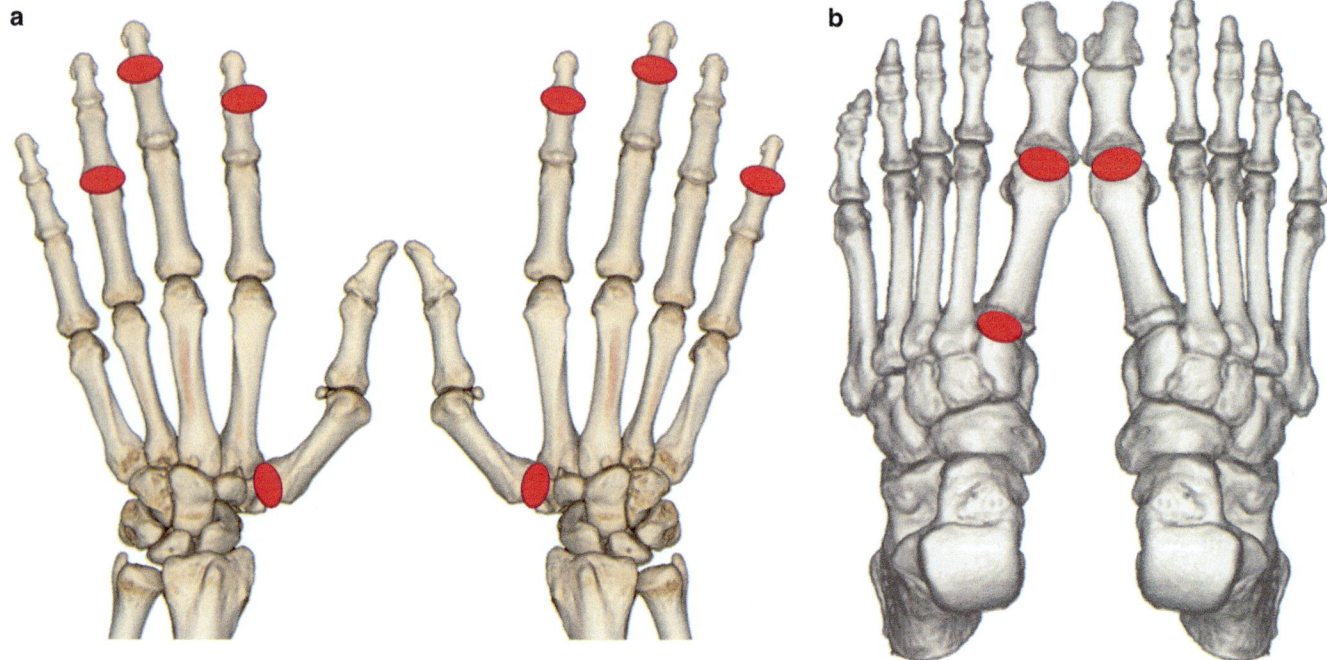

Fig. 1 Primary osteoarthritis, seat of the lesions: diagram of hands (**a**) and feet (**b**), dorsal view. Bilateral and relatively symmetrical polyarthropathy: note the prevalent involvement of the DIP, the scarcity of the involvement of the MCP, and the prevalent involvement of the first toe

the PIP (+), and of the carpometacarpal joint of the thumb (++: rhizarthrosis). Rarely impacts MCP

- Foot: tarsometatarsal articulation (first ray ++), MTP (first ray ++: hallux rigidus) (Fig. 1)

Paraclinical examination:

- Lab tests: Normal ESR and PCR
- **X-ray**: evaluate using "**ONSC**" criteria (mnemotechnic means to remember the order of appearance of the radiological lesions)
  - **O**steophytes at the joint margin.
  - **N**arrowing joint: asymmetrical, compared to the weight-bearing area.
  - Subchondral **S**clerosis.
  - Subchondral **C**yst.
  - N.B.: Narrowing can occur before the osteophytes in certain articulations.
- ArthroCT: very powerful but seldom necessary, evaluates "ONSC" criteria
  - And assesses cartilage precisely:
    Thickness.
    Search for microfractures
    The cartilage is a low-density tissue between two structures of high density (intra-articular contrast agent and subchondral bone plate).
- Bone scan:
  - Is positive during the active phase of osteoarthritis

- MRI:
  - To evaluate the cartilage
  - And the subchondral osseous edema

Differential:

- Inflammatory rheumatism
- Fracture
- Synostosis (Fig. 2)

Classification: Table 1 [61, 63]

- Kellgren and Lawrence [63]:
  - For knee osteoarthritis.
  - Knee osteoarthritis is classified into five radiological stages, by taking into account the osteophytes and the articular narrowing.
- Modified Kellgren and Lawrence [61]:
  - Adapted to all the sites of osteoarthritis

Evolution:

- Progressive aggravation, in general slow with inflammatory phase of effusion (hydrarthrosis).
- Existence of a few quickly evolving forms (rapidly destructive coxarthrosis).

Fig. 2 Intermetatarsal M3-M4 evolutive osteoarthritis of the right foot, plantar blood pool phase (**a**) and fused transverse slice (**b**). Not to confuse with intermetatarsal synostosis (rare pathology, young subjects, osseous bridge visible on CT)

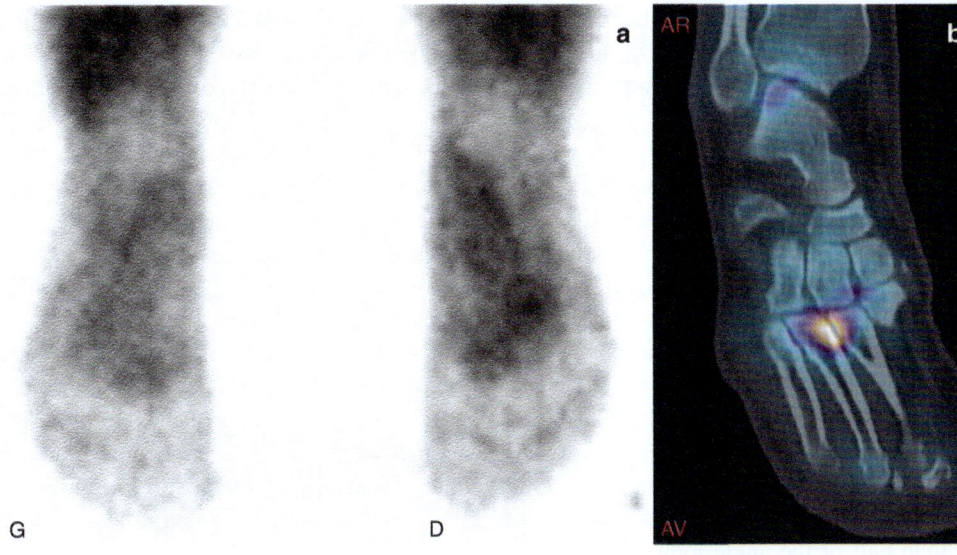

Table 1 Osteoarthritis: grades and radiological classifications

Grade	0	I	II	III	IV
Classification	Normal	Doubtful	Minimal	Moderate	Severe
According to Kellgren and Lawrence (for the knee only)					
Description	No sign of osteoarthritis	Minimal osteophytes of uncertain significance	Visible osteophytes, no joint space narrowing	Visible osteophytes, moderate joint space narrowing	Severe joint space narrowing, subchondral bone sclerosis
According to modified Kellgren and Lawrence (for all joints)					
O	–	Possible onset	Visible	Visible	Frank
N	–	Doubtful	Visible	Visible	Severe
S	–	–	–	Beginning	Severe
C	–	–	–	–	Visible

O osteophytes, **N** narrowing joint, **S** subchondral sclerosis, **C** subchondral cyst

Treatment [12]:

- **Symptomatic:**
  - Decrease modifiable RF: **weight loss** (+++), orthopedic soles, etc.
  - **Physical exercise:** adapted, movement is part of osteoarthritis treatment and makes it possible to decrease pain and disability.
    General (+++): gym, fitness
    And local (+++): muscular and neuromuscular reinforcement
  - Drugs per os:
    Fast action: **paracetamol** (+++), NSAIDs, weak opioids
    Slow action: sulfate chondroitin, glucosamine, unsaponifiables (not of notable effectiveness compared to placebo [64])
  - Intra-articular drugs:
    Fast action: corticoids (if severe and inflammatory osteoarthritis)
    Slow action: hyaluronic acid (= viscosupplementation)
- Curative: prosthesis

Discussion:

- Delayed bone scan imaging is **positive** during the **active** osteoarthritis phase. In the event of radiological osteoarthritis, the absence of uptake testifies to the stable nature of the pathology and eliminates an evolutive osteoarthritis [61].
- A study of 20 patients evaluated the inter- and intra-observer reproducibility of examinations to localize evolutive osteoarthritis of the ankle and foot: the bone SPECT-CT has perfect inter- and intra-observer reproducibility, significantly higher than the CT alone, than

planar bone scan alone and than coupled reading of planar bone scans and CT. Bone SPECT-CT is a very good examination to locate osteoarthritis precisely to be treated by infiltration or arthrodesis [66].

- A study of bone SPECT-CT on 27 patients suffering from deformation of the back of the foot and ankle deformation found that the signs of osteoarthritis prevail on the medial part of the ankle in the event of varus deformations and on the lateral part in the event of valgus deformations. Bone SPECT-CT allows a precise and very early visualization of these modifications, independently of the clinical degree of deformation, and can be a decision-making for realignment osteotomy [66]. Ankle osteoarthritis is post-traumatic in 80% of the cases and is readily asymmetrical, following poor ankle alignment. Among young patients with moderate asymmetrical osteoarthritis, where more than half of the ankle joint surface is preserved, realignment surgery via supra-malleolar osteotomy could be the more adapted Tx: bone SPECT-CT can be very useful in specifying the exact ankle osteoarthritis topography and to assess the state of nearby articulations [67].

- A retrospective study was carried out among 50 patients suffering from foot and ankle pain with an uncertain final diagnosis, in spite of a clinical examination by an orthopedist specialist in the foot and ankle and standard radiographies: the initial diagnosis agreed with bone SPECT-CT in 22% of the cases. In 78% of the patients (39/50), the results disagreed, and the SPECT-CT anomalies led to a modification of care for all patients, with an improvement of the symptoms in 76% of the patients (38/50): the diagnostic performance of the bone SPECT-CT is excellent (94%) and particularly useful in the event of osteoarthritis of both the front and back of the foot [36].

- Another retrospective study related on 86 patients with ankle and foot pain without certain diagnoses after specialized clinical examination, standard radiographies, and more or fewer other examinations (ultrasound, CT, MRI): bone SPECT-CT led to a change in the initial diagnosis and Tx in 69% of the patients (59/86). Ninety-three percent of the patients (80/86) had improvement of symptoms after a Tx based on the results of SPECT-CT. The authors signal that these patients with hard-to-analyze foot pain only represent 10% of the patients treated for the same period in their specialized ankle and foot orthopedic service [68].

- An exploratory study on 30 patients suffering from chronic pain of the foot showed the feasibility of antalgic infiltration guided by diagnostic CT on the articular or peri-osseous zones with the most uptake on the bone SPECT-CT. 90% of the patients (27/30) had an improvement of the symptoms, in particular 93% of the patients suffering from osteoarthritis (13/14) and 100% of the patients suffering from OLT (10/10). The bone SPECT-CT led to a modification of the foreseeable site of injection in 53% of the patients (16/30) and in particular in 100% of the patients presenting a pain of forefoot (9/9) [69].

Box 1

Osteoarthritis: modifiable risk factors

- Obesity (+++)
- Axial disorders
- Repeated trauma (sport, work)

Box 2

Pain is not correlated with the radiological importance of osteoarthritis [62] but is correlated with the activity on bone SPECT-CT [65, 70]. Moreover bone SPECT-CT has a strong negative predictive value regarding the progression of osteoarthritis [71].

Osteoarthritis of the Foot: Common Localization

Primary Osteoarthritis (Fig. 3, Table 2)

Hallux rigidus (osteoarthritis of the MTP of the first ray) [6, 21, 42]:

- Second most frequent affection of the MTP of the first ray after the hallux valgus
- Clinical examination:
  - Mechanical pain on the dorsal surface of the MTP
  - **Increases when stepping**
  - Impingement due to the dorsal osteophytes:
    With the shoe/extensor of the first toe
  - Sometimes misleading signs in the event of antalgic reflex supination with:
    Overload of the fifth ray (sometimes as far as fracture)
    Or tenosynovitis of the tibialis posterior

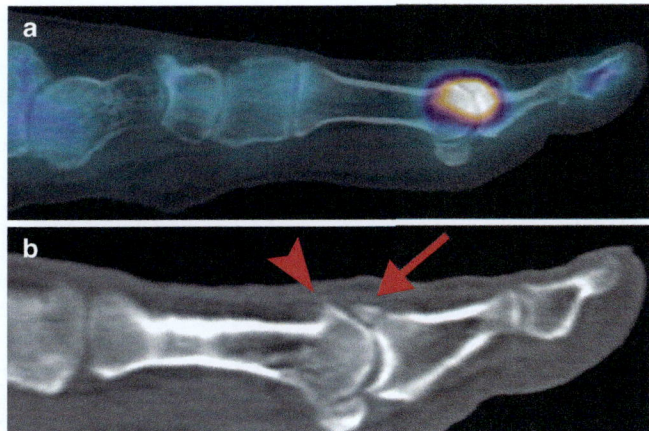

Fig. 4 Hallux rigidus, sagittal fused (**a**) and CT (**b**) slices. The osteoarthritis of the MTP of the first ray is usually primary: it is secondary here to an old injury, with sequela of a bone tear at the base of P1 (arrow). Note the dorsal osteophyte (arrow head)

- Etiology:
  - Often primary
  - +/− secondary:
    Mechanical overload (excess length of M1 or P1)
    Traumatic antecedents, osteochondritis (Fig. 4)
- Evolution:
  - Compensation with antalgic supination and overload on M5
  - Ankylosis
- Tx:
  - Medical: adapted shoes, soles, etc.
  - Surgery:
    Dorsal osteophytes: resection
    Osteotomy, arthrodesis

Tarsometatarsal osteoarthritis [17, 42]:

- Prevails on the **medial side** between the medial cuneiform and M1 (= rhizarthrosis of the foot) (Fig. 5)
- Clinical examination:
  - Pain upon pressure and mobilization of the tarsometatarsal articulation
  - Impingement with shoes due to the dorsal osteophytes
- Etiology:
  - Can be primary
  - Often secondary:
    Prior tarsal injury
    Foot stress disorder: flatfoot with valgus of the back part of the foot and overload on the medial longitudinal arch
    Hallux valgus
- Can be associated with proximal involvement of talocalcaneonavicular and cuneonavicular joints

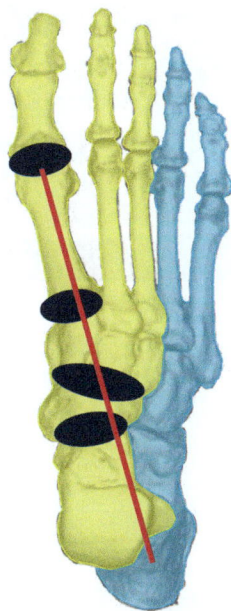

Fig. 3 Medial longitudinal arch and most frequent topography of primary osteoarthritis of the foot: diagram of the foot, dorsal view. Red feature: medial longitudinal arch. In black: osteoarthritis. In yellow: propelling talar foot. In blue: calcaneal support foot

Table 2 Osteoarthritis of the foot: most frequent location

Joint	Medial/lateral side	Frequency
Metatarsophalangeal	Medial: first ray (hallux rigidus)	≈60% of foot osteoarthritis
Tarsometatarsal	Medial: first ray	≈15%
Transverse tarsal	Medial: talocalcaneonavicular and cuneonavicular	≈10%

N. B. Osteoarthritis of the foot primarily impacts the joints of the **medial longitudinal arch**, because they are the most called upon for propulsion

Fig. 5 Bilateral medial tarsometatarsal osteoarthritis, front view of WB (**a**), fused transverse (**b**), and sagittal (**c**) slices. 65-year-old man, left hip pain increasing over the past 5 months: left superolateral coxarthrosis and focal uptake of the anterior femoral neck more evocative of a stress fracture than of an anterior impingement in this patient (SPECT-CT not shown). Note the bilateral evolutive osteoarthritis of the hands and feet: carpometacarpal osteoarthritis of the thumb (rhizarthrosis, between the trapezium and M1) and medial tarsometatarsal osteoarthritis (rhizarthrosis of the foot, between the medial cuneiform and M1)

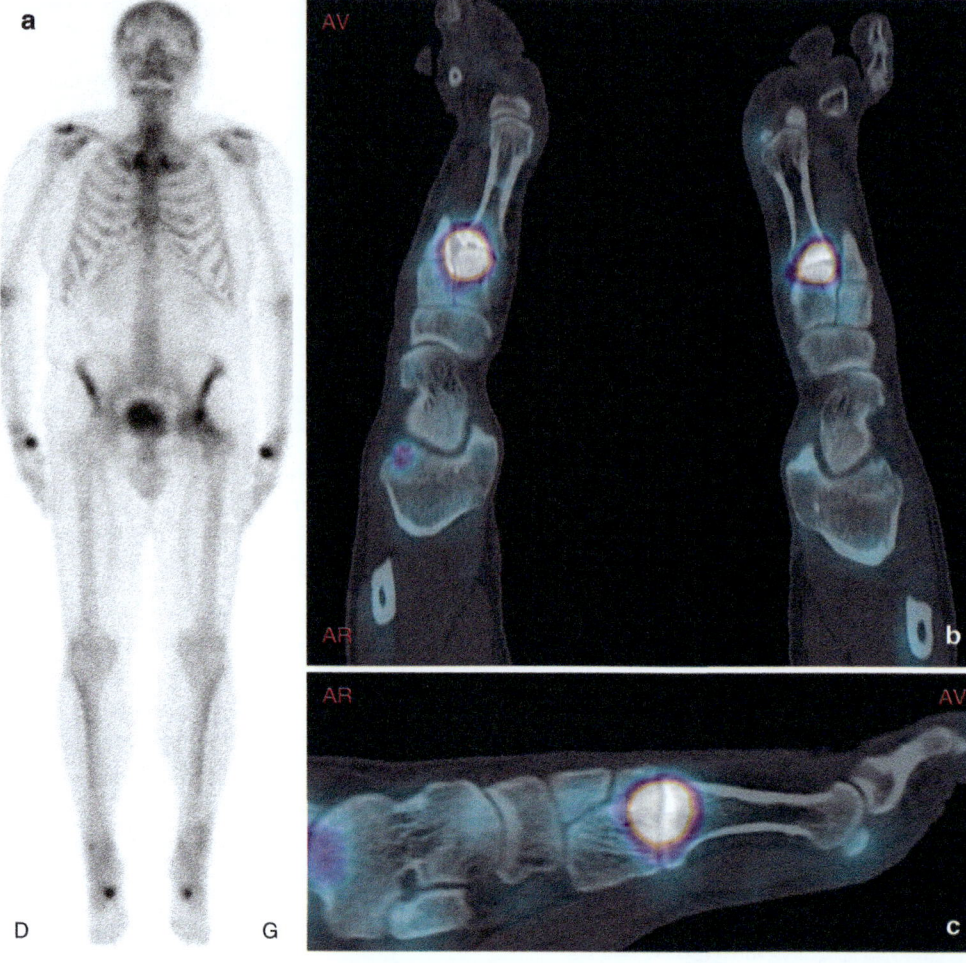

- Tx:
  - Medical (+++): soles and infiltration
  - Surgery:
    Dorsal osteophytes: resection
    Arthrodesis

Secondary Osteoarthritis

Osteoarthritis of the transverse tarsal joint [17]:

- Prevalent on the **medial side** between the talus and the navicular (and between the navicular and the three cunei-forms) (Fig. 6)
- Clinical examination:
  - Pain upon pressure and with mobilization of the transverse tarsal joint
  - Impingement with shoes due to the dorsal osteophytes
- Etiology:
  - Often secondary: idem osteoarthritis of the tarsometatarsal joints (Fig. 7)
- Tx: idem osteoarthritis of the tarsometatarsal joints

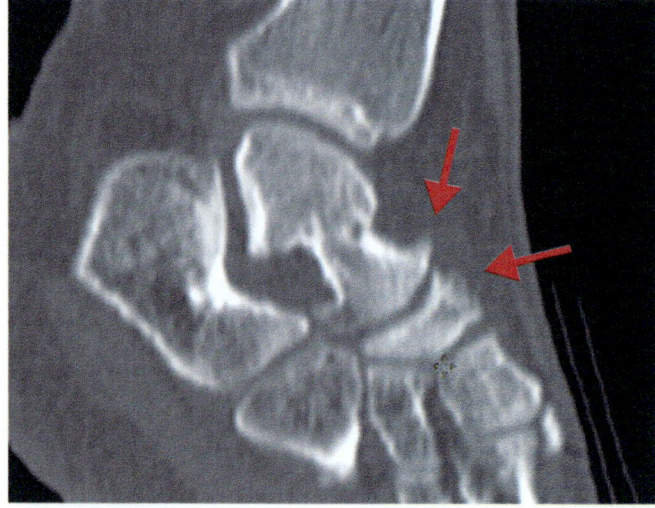

Fig. 6 Talocalcaneonavicular osteoarthritis, sagittal CT slice. Note the dorsal osteophytes (arrows)

Subtalar osteoarthritis [21]:

- Clinical examination:
  - Lateral submalleolar mechanical pain
  - Pain with **walking on rough ground** (forced eversion-inversion)

Fig. 7 Calcaneocuboid osteoarthritis post-fracture of the cuboid, front view of WB (**a**), sagittal CT (**b**), and fused (**c**) slices. 17-year-old girl, right cuboid fracture 2 years ago, treated by bone graft 1 year ago: persistence of pain. Note that the very focal articular uptake is almost not discernible on the WB

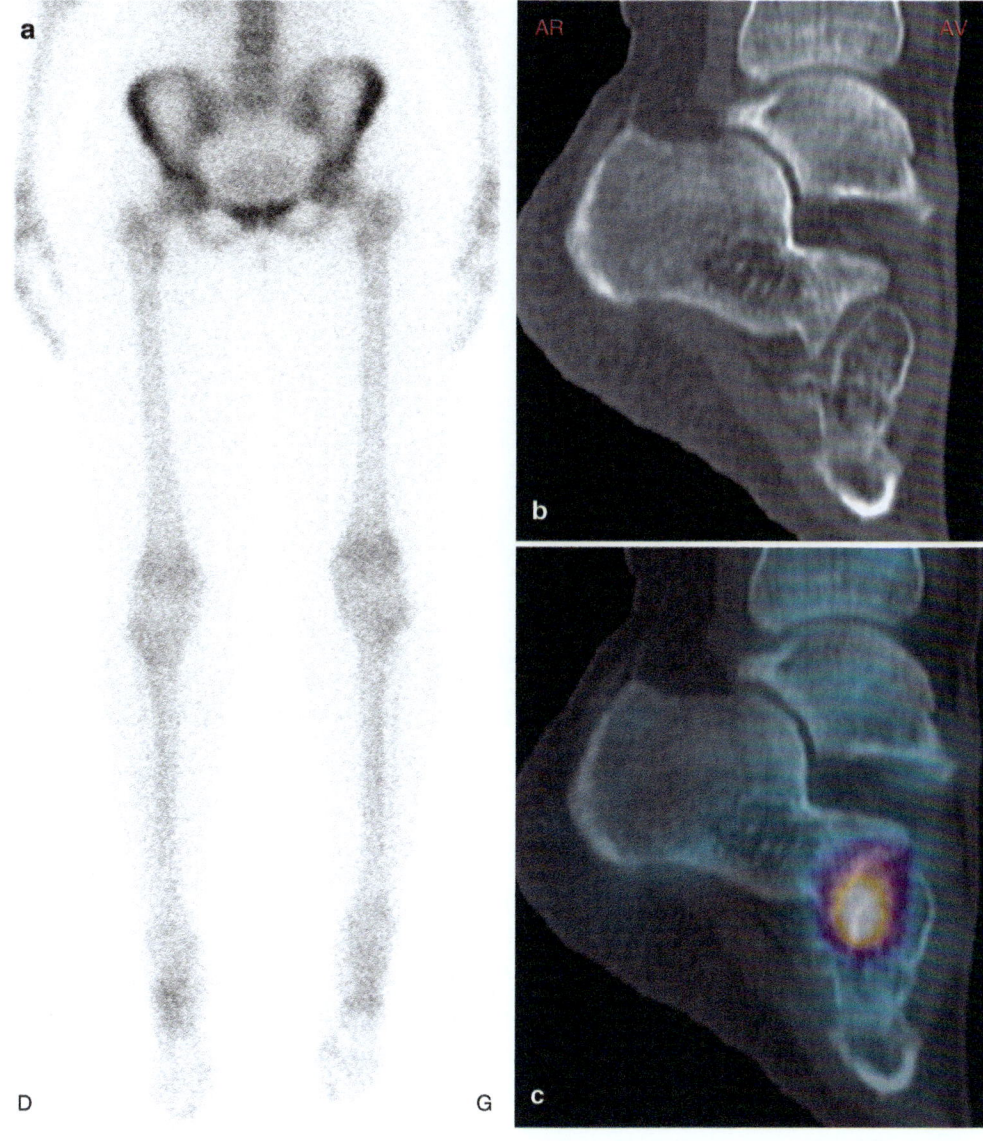

- Etiology:
  - Orientation disorder of the back foot
  - Prior trauma: **calcaneal fracture** (Fig. 8)
- Differential: ankle osteoarthritis
- Tx:
  - Medical: soles and infiltration
  - Surgery:
    Subtalar arthrodesis (+++)

Ankle osteoarthritis [21]:

- Clinical examination:
  - Mechanical pain of ankle (on the level of the anterior line space)

  - **Loss of foot flexion**
  - Swelling
- Etiology:
  - Prior trauma:
    Bimalleolar fracture
    Repeated **sprains** with OLT
- Differential: subtalar osteoarthritis
- Tx:
  - Medical:
    Viscosupplementation, chondroprotectors, soles
  - Surgery:
    Arthrodesis of the ankle
    Total ankle prosthesis [17]

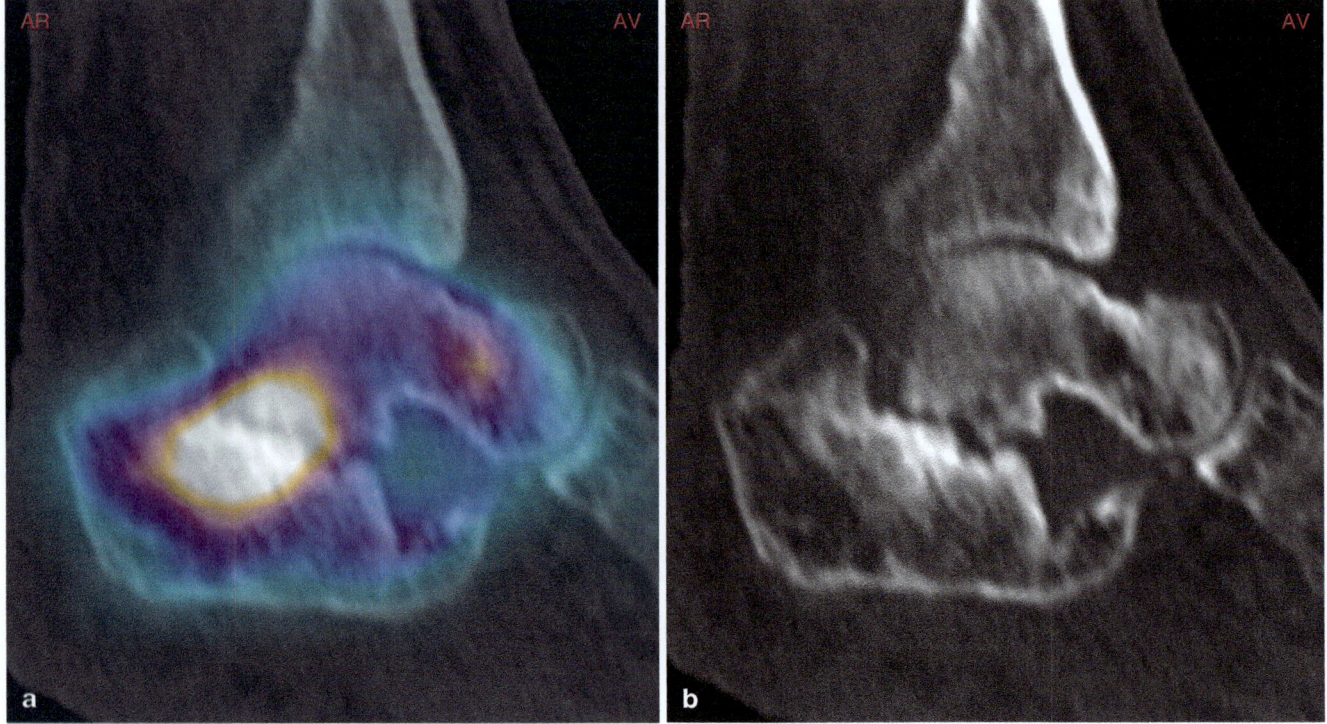

Fig. 8 (**a** and **b**) Subtalar osteoarthritis subsequent to a fracture of the calcaneus 10 months prior, sagittal fused (**a**) and CT (**b**) slices

Box 3
Soccer foot [17]:
   Solicitation of feet in movement and kicks (microtrauma)
   After 20 years of practice:

- Osteoarthritis:
  – Very frequent (60% of the subjects) of which:
    Talocalcaneonavicular (20%)
    Ankle (15%)
  – Often not very symptomatic
  – X-ray, "ONSC" signs:
    Osteophytes: many and exuberant
    Narrowing: absent, preserved space
- Anterior and posterior impingement

Rheumatoid Arthritis (RA)

Predisposition [42, 72]:

- **Women** (M/F = 1/3)
- Between 40 and 60 years of age

Past medical history: NR
Frequency [72]:

- **Frequent**
- Prevalence: 0.5–1%

Mechanism [61]:

- There is citrullination (transformation of the amino acid arginine into citrulline) followed by immunization (auto-immune response to citrullinated peptides): the immune system produces autoantibodies against the antigens via the activation of T lymphocytes and then synoviocytes. Synovitis follows, with production of proteolytic enzymes and factors promoting the bone resorption (TNF +++), followed by osteocartilaginous destruction.
- 50% of risk of developing RA is attributable to genetic factors [72].

Types [61]:

- Early stage (the first 6–12 months):
  - Synovitis without irreversible lesions
- End stage:
  - Irreversible osteoarticular lesions
  - Extra-articular manifestations

Interview [61]:

- Distal oligoarthritis or polyarthritis (70%) (Fig. 9):
  - **Inflammatory arthritis**:
    Bilateral and **symmetrical**
    Of the **wrists**, the hands (second or third **MCP** and **PIP**) or of the feet (**MTP**) (Fig. 10)
  - Morning stiffness of inflammatory nature, lasting longer than 15 min (different from osteoarthritis)
  - Discrete CIC, fever = 38°
  - Begins progressively
- Feverish acute polyarthritis (20%):
  - Idem distal polyarthritis
  - CIC (+++), fever >38.5°
  - Begins suddenly
- Other articular manifestations (10%):
  - Rhizomelic attack (shoulders, hips)

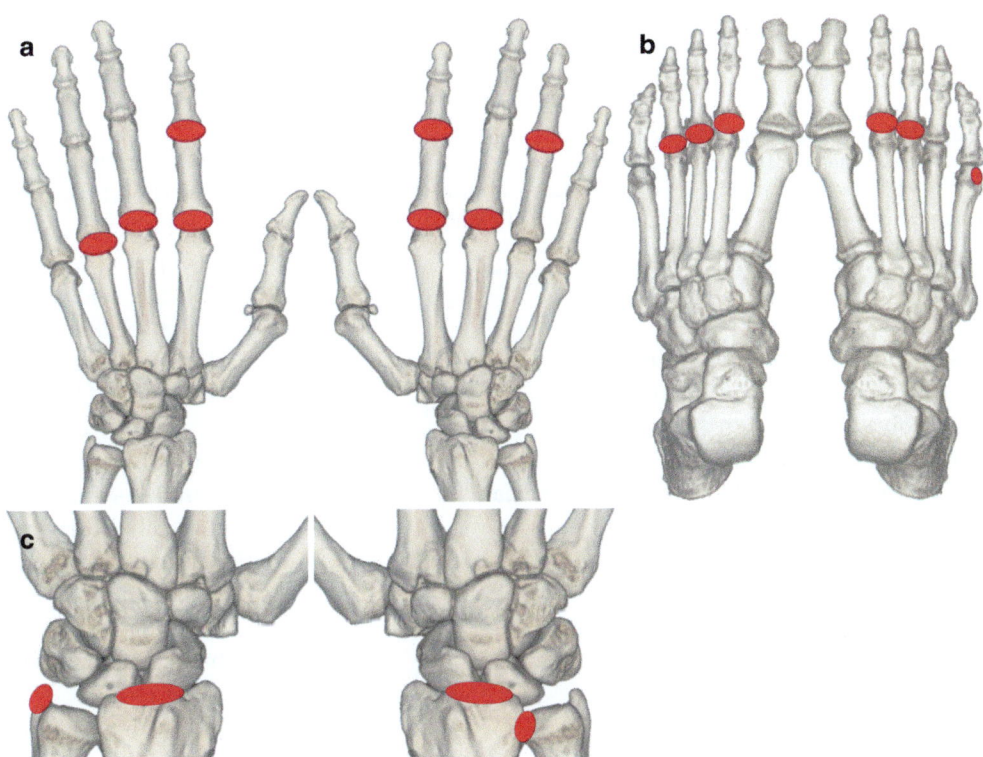

Fig. 9 Rheumatoid arthritis, synovitis, and bone erosion sites: diagram of the hands (**a**), feet (**b**), and wrists (**c**), dorsal view. Bilateral and symmetrical arthritis: note the involvement of the wrists, the MCP/MTP, PIP, and the respect of the DIP

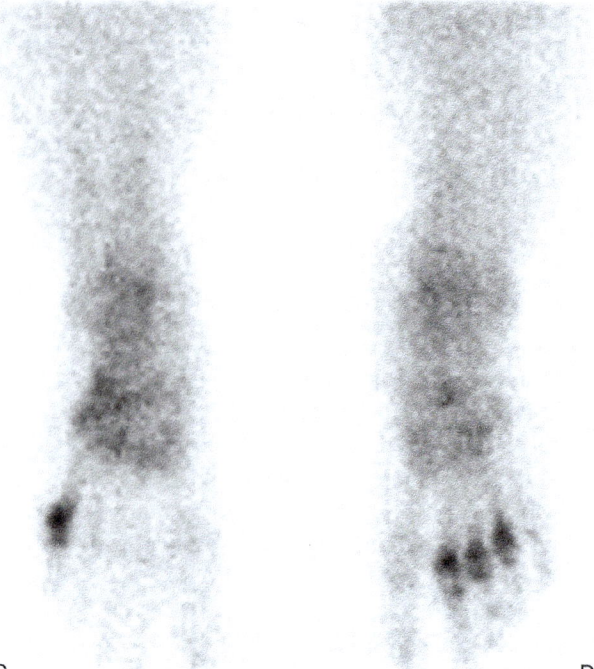

G   D

Fig. 10 Rheumatoid arthritis, osteoarticular lesions of the MTP: plantar delayed image

Table 3 Rheumatoid arthritis: location of early lesions

	Synovitis	Bone destruction
Wrist	Wrist joint Distal radioulnar	Ulnar styloid process +/− capitate, lunate, triquetrum, scaphoid
Hand	MCP (+++, especially second and third) PIP (more moderate)	Radial edge of the heads of M2 and M3 Ulnar edge of the head of M5
Feet	MTP (+++) +/− IP of the hallux	Lateral edge of the head of M5 +/− posterior part of the calcaneal tuberosity

- Chronic monoarthritis (wrist, knee)
- Intermittent mono−/oligoarthritis
- Polyarthralgia
• Frequent tenosynovitis
• Extra-articular manifestations (rarely indicative):
  - Rheumatoid vascularitis
  - Pleuropulmonary impairment
  - Rheumatoid nodules

Clinical examination [61]:

• Early stage:
  - Arthritis:
    Painful articular swelling with stiffness and local inflammatory signs
    Hands, wrists, and feet (Table 3)

• End stage:
  - Articular deformations of the hands, wrists, and feet
  - Cervical spine impairment:
    High neck pain, frequent
    C1-C2 luxation: synovitis with periodontoid pannus; rarer with therapeutic advances
  - Appendicular articulations impairment: shoulders, elbows, knees, ankles, hips
  - Rheumatoid nodules:
    ≤1 cm
    Subcutaneous (seldom visceral)
    Upper limbs: forearm, elbows, hands
  - Systemic manifestations:
    Pleuropulmonary: pleurisy, fibrosis, nodules
    Cardiovascular: primarily due to the chronic systemic inflammation
  - Rheumatoid vasculitis:
    By deposits of immune complexes
    Late, seldom symptomatic

Paraclinical examinations:

• Lab tests [61]:
  - ESR and CRP ↗
  - Rheumatoid factor (RF), anti-IgG Ab:
    Often negative during early stage
    Very often positive after 6 months of evolution
    Nonspecific
  - Anti-citrullinated peptide Ab (ACPA):
    Often positive during early stage
    Very specific
  - Antinuclear antibodies (ANA):
    Can be slightly positive
    Anti-dsDNA Ab, specific to lupus, is generally negative
• X-rays [42]:
  - Feet, hands, and wrists, systematic
  - Look for specific lesions:
    Early: tumefaction, strips of osseous rarefaction in MCP and MTP (especially fifth MTP)
    Late: osseous erosion (ulnar styloid process, lateral edge of the fifth metatarsal head)
• **Ultrasound** (+++) [42]:
  - Can visualize early lesions well
  - Feet, hands, and wrists
  - Articular effusion, **synovitis**
  - Tenosynovitis
  - Sub- and intermetatarsal bursitis
  - Osseous erosion
• MRI (++) with gadolinium IV [42]:
  - Hand and wrist the most symptomatic
  - Idem ultrasound
  - + **Bone marrow edema** (sign appearing earlier than bone erosion and is reversible)

Differential [61]:

- Monoarthritis: septic, microcrystalline (gout)
- Oligo–/polyarthritis:
  - Septic
  - Spondylarthropathy
  - Polymyalgia rheumatica (PMR): inflammatory rheumatism most frequent in older subjects, impacting shoulders and hips
  - Systemic lupus erythematosus (SLE): 10 times rarer than RA, younger women

Classification [61, 72]:

- ACR criteria revised in 1987: do not allow early diagnosis
- ACR/EULAR 2010 criteria: allows early diagnosis, classification currently used (Table 4) [61, 72, 73]

Treatment [21, 42, 61]:

- Therapeutic urgency: there is a therapeutic window during which it is possible to obtain remission and optimal control
- **Early Tx**, within 3 months, in order to:
  - Resolve synovites
  - Delay the appearance of bone erosion (irreversible)
- Symptomatic Tx = conventional Tx
  - Analgesics, NSAIDs, corticoids (++)

Table 4 ACR/EULAR 2010 rheumatoid arthritis criteria. Faced with a beginning polyarthritis with normal X-rays and without a diagnosis of any other disease

	Score
Joint involvement	(0–5)
– 1 large joint	0
– 2–10 large joints	1
– 1–3 small joints	2
– 4–10 small joints	3
– >10 joints (including at least 1 small)	5
Serology	(0–3)
– Negative RF and negative ACPA	0
– Low positive RF (1–3× the normal) or low positive ACPA (1–3× the normal)	2
– High positive RF (>3× normal) or high positive ACPA (>3× the normal)	3
Acute-phase reactants	(0–1)
– Normal ESR and normal CRP	0
– Abnormal ESR or abnormal CRP	1
Duration of the symptoms	(0–1)
– <6 weeks	0
– ≥6 weeks	1
A score ≥ 6 classifies the patient as having RA	

- Basic Tx = disease-modifying antirheumatic drugs (DMARDs):
  - **Methotrexate** (+++)
  - Leflunomide (Arava), sulfasalazine
  - Biotherapies: **anti-TNF-α** (+++, Remicade, Enbrel)

Evolution [61]:

- **Successive periods of exacerbation and lesions worsen**:
  - Quickly evolving serious form (10%)
  - Traditional form with major disability at 10 years (50%)
  - Benign form with little discomfort at 10 years (25%)
- Lulls/remissions between the periods of exacerbation
- The severity of rheumatoid arthritis might be lessening, with improved disease outcome, and better Tx seems the dominant factor (both conventional Tx and DMARDs) [72]

Discussion:

- In the event of suspicion of RA in the clinical examination, the bone scan should systematically include blood pool imaging of the hands (palmar) and feet (plantar). These images could be the only ones to be positive during the early stage (synovitis without bone erosion). This is the same for suspicion of psoriatic arthritis, where there is a peripheral joint involvement. In case of suspicion of ankylosing spondylitis, pelvic-lumbar blood pool images are usually non-conclusive because vascular (common iliac vessels) and urinary (ureter) activities impede the imaging: therefore, we systematically realize blood pool imaging of the hands and feet and a sacroiliac joint or a lumbar inflammation will be looked for on the delayed images with SPECT-CT. For all these reasons, in the event of suspicion of inflammatory rheumatism, we almost always perform plantar and palmar blood pool imaging, because of their high diagnostic impact and because they could be the only images to be positive in case of RA (the most frequent inflammatory rheumatism).
- An early diagnosis of RA allows early treatment with DMARDs (in the first 3 months) and a major reduction in functional impotence [42]. The ACR/EULAR 2010 RA criteria make it possible to diagnose early stage RA to begin quick treatment [72].
- A study compared bone scan (BS) and the 2010 ACR/EULAR criteria for RA diagnosis in a group of 75 patients with arthritis, including 56 with RA as a final diagnosis. The BS is not useful in the event of score ≥ 6: the BS has a Se and Sp of, respectively, 80% (45/56) and 79% (15/19), and the 2010 ACR/EULAR classification criteria have Se and Sp of, respectively, 82% (46/56) and 95% (18/19). The authors also assess the usefulness of a

composite classification, a bone scan-assisted 2010 criteria, with which the number and the topography of hyperactivity in the blood pool images of BS were used as reference for calculating articular impairment in the 2010 ACR/EULAR criteria: in the event of 2010 criteria <6 (28 patients including 10 with RA), the BS-assisted 2010 criteria had a better sensitivity of 30%(3/10) vs 0% at the price of a slight reduction in Sp, with 95% (17/18) vs 100%. According to authors, this BS-assisted 2010 classification could also be useful for patients for whom clinical articular examination is difficult, particularly those already using anti-inflammatory medication [74].

Box 4
Rheumatoid arthritis:

The most frequent inflammatory rheumatism
Women between 40 and 60 years of age
Bilateral and symmetrical polyarthritis
Impacting the wrists, MCP, PIP, and MTP

Box 5
The foot is impacted in more than 80% of RA cases [21, 42].

Foot impairment is inaugural in 10–25% of RA cases [21].

Box 6
In the event of scintigraphic RA suspicion, nuclear physicians should make sure the patient sees a rheumatologist within 2 weeks.

Psoriatic Arthritis

Definition:

- Peripheral spondyloarthritis associated with cutaneous psoriasis

Predisposition [61, 75]:

- 30–50 years of age
- Ratio M/F = 1

Past medical history [61]:

- **Psoriasis** (by definition):
  - Especially of the nails, of the folds (inverse psorisasis), or of the scalp
  - Whatever the extent of the psoriasis
  - Present before or at the moment of the diagnosis in 85% of cases
  - Can occur after the rheumatologic manifestations in ≈15% of cases [76]
- Genetic factors: **HLA** B27 or B39 or Cw6, +/− psoriatic arthritis in a first-degree relative

Frequency [61, 75]:

- **Frequent**
- Prevalence ≈ 0.2%

Mechanism:

- Auto-inflammation: microtrauma to the joints and entheses are responsible for repeated micro-lesions and repairs, with chronic regional micro-inflammation and a poorly adapted immune response in subjects with genetic predisposition [61]. It results in a proliferation of T CD8 lymphocytes and secretion of cytokines, interferon, and TNF-α in the joints (synovial membrane and synovial fluid) and the entheses, causing **arthritis** and **enthesitis** [61]. The zones of enthesitis are related to **osseous erosion**, which heal in the form of fibrosis with characteristic **progressive ossification**, responsible for enthesophytes (vertebral syndesmophytes, calcaneal enthesophytes, etc.) [41]. The progression of the enthesophytes is responsible for articular stiffness: **ankylosis**, more frequent in the ankylosing spondylitis than in psoriatic arthritis.

Types: NR

Interview and clinical examination [21, 61]:

- **Impairment of peripheral articulations > axial articulations**
- Peripheral articular impairment:
  - **Asymmetrical oligoarthritis/monoarthritis** (70%) (Fig. 11):
    Of the **lower limbs: knee, foot**
    +/− Wrist
  - Symmetrical polyarthritis (20%): can look like RA
  - Impairment of one or more **DIP** (Fig. 12):
    Isolated (5%) or associated other articular impairment
    Very evocative
- Axial articular impairment:
  - Touches 25% of patients at time of diagnosis and up to 50% of the patients during the course of the disease [76]
  - Especially on the **cervical rachis**
  - May be revealing: psoriatic pelvic spondylitis (5%)
- **Enthesitis** (+++):
  - Touches more than 30% of patients during the course of their disease [76]
  - Inferior limbs: **calcaneus** (+++) posterior (calcaneal tendon) or plantar (plantar aponeurosis), responsible for **posterior talalgia**

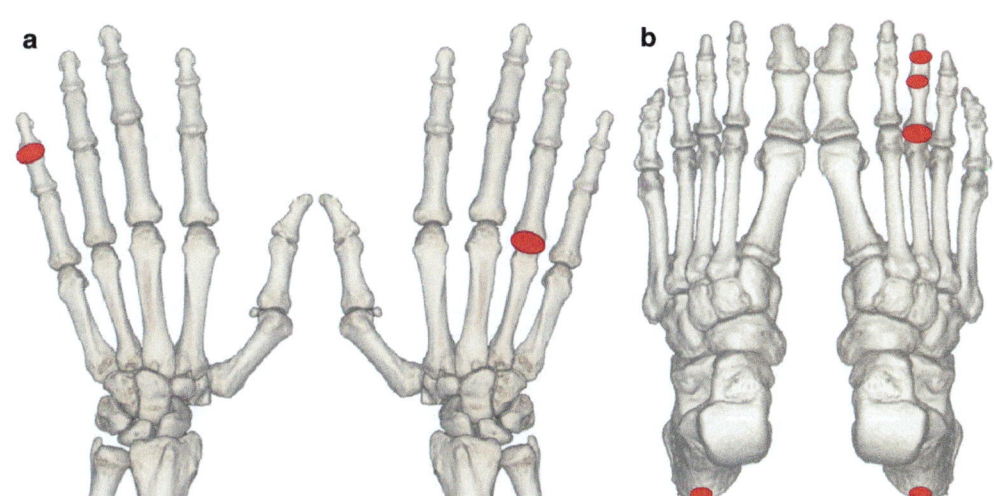

Fig. 11 Psoriatic arthritis, lesions sites: diagram of the hands (**a**) and feet (**b**), dorsal view. Asymmetrical oligoarthritis: note involvement of the DIP, the possible radiate involvement (MCP/MTP + PIP + DIP), and the calcaneal enthesitis

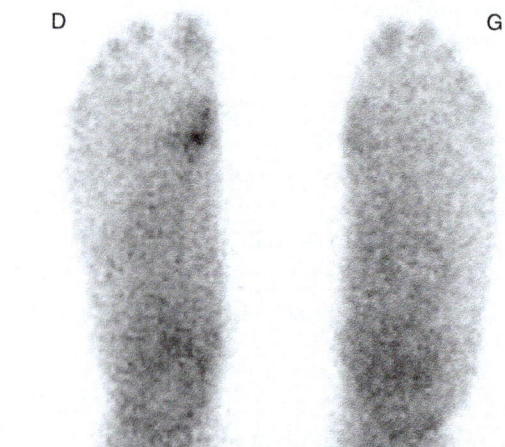

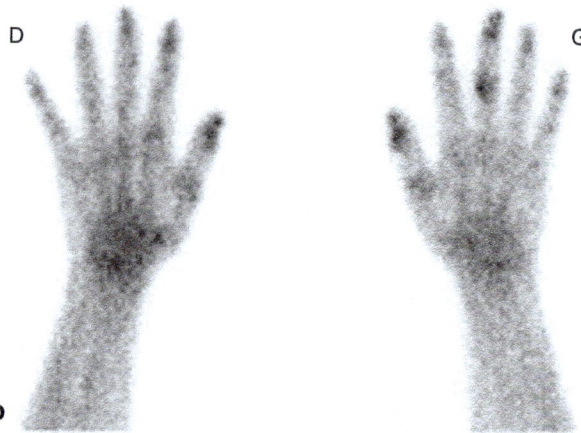

Fig. 12 Psoriatic arthritis of the hands and the feet, delayed plantar (**a**) and palmar (**b**) images. 50-year-old woman, antecedents of guttate psoriasis 15 years ago: suspicion of psoriatic arthritis in view of diffuse articular pain for the past 6 weeks predominantly in the hands, wrists, shoulders, spine, and feet. On bone scan, asymmetrical oligoarthropa- thy of the feet and hands: note involvement of a DIP (third ray of the left hand and probably second and third rays on the right), quasi-radial involvement (third ray of the left hand), and probable involvement of the right wrist. No other lesion on the whole body (images not shown). Psoriatic arthritis confirmed afterward

- **Dactylitis** (+++):
  - Touches up to 50% of patients during the course of their disease and is associated with the increased risk of bone erosion [76]
  - **Radial** involvement:
    Pandactylitis with involvement of a whole ray (MTP-PIP-DIP or MCP-PIP-DIP).
    Tumefaction of a finger or a toe ("sausage toe")
  - Painful or not
  - Rather evocative
- Synovitis, bursitis, tenosynovitis:
  - Rather evocative of an inflammatory pathology
  - Bursitis can erode the bone, particularly with the calcaneus (can also be seen in the event of RA) [42] (Fig. 13)
- Systemic involvement (not very frequent):
  - Ocular: uveitis, conjunctivitis
  - Cardiac: aortic insufficiency
  - Cardiovascular complications: due to chronic systemic inflammation inducing atheromatosis

Paraclinical examinations:

- Lab tests [61]:
  - ESR and CRP:
    Can be ↗ during periods of exacerbation, but much less often than with RA
    Normal results do not eliminate the diagnosis
  - Rheumatoid factor: often negative
  - HLA B27 (or B39 or Cw6) often positive

- **X-rays** (+++):
  - Hands and feet
    Looking for arthritis and hyperostotic erosion
  - Sacroiliac and rachis
- Ultrasound:
  - Hands and feet
  - Looking for **enthesitis**, synovitis, tenosynovitis
- **MRI**:
  - Of a hand or a foot:
    Look for arthritis, synovitis, enthesitis, bursitis
    And **bone edema** in view of enthesitis, extensive
  - Sacroiliac and rachis

Differential:

- Rheumatoid arthritis:
  - ≈ as frequent, ≈ same age
  - Women
  - Positive rheumatoid factor
  - **No involvement of the DIP**
  - Symmetrical polyarthritis of MCP/MTP and PIP
- Mechanical enthesopathy of the calcaneus:
  - Enthesophytes of the plantar aponeurosis and the calcaneal tendon are very frequent, in particular in athletes, and the various types of imagery cannot differentiate them from a rheumatic enthesitis [42].

Classification:

- CASPAR (2006) criteria: specificity, 91.4%, and Sp, 98.7%, for a dg of psoriatic arthritis (Table 5) [61, 77] (Table 6) [61, 75] and (Table 7)

Fig. 13 Right posterior talalgia: pre-tendinous erosive bursitis, posterior view of WB (**a**), sagittal fused (**b**), and CT (**c**) slices. The analysis of the WB could make one think of an aspecific calcaneal enthesopathy: the SPECT-CT shows that site of intense uptake does not correspond to the zone where the calcaneal tendon embeds but is above it, in front of the synovial bursa of calcaneal tendon and corresponds to small bone erosion on the CT, in connection with spondyloarthritis in this 70-year-old man followed for Crohn's colitis

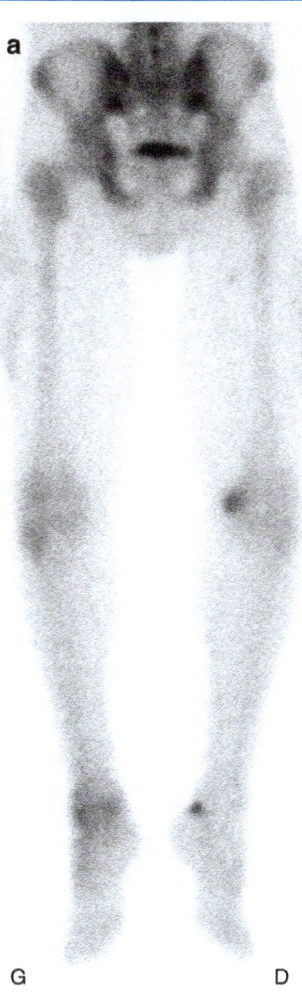

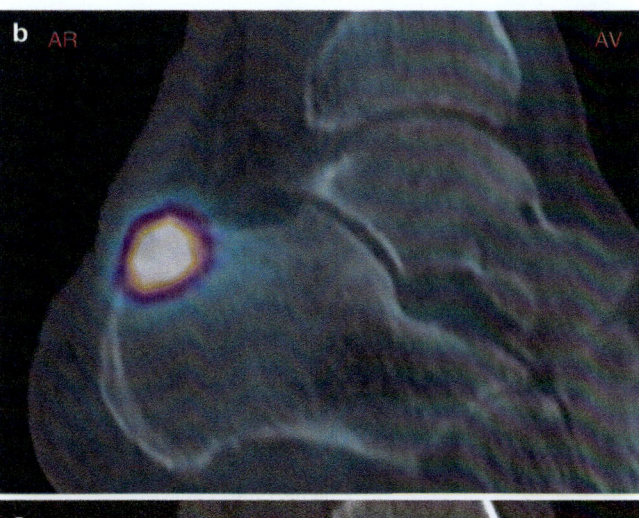

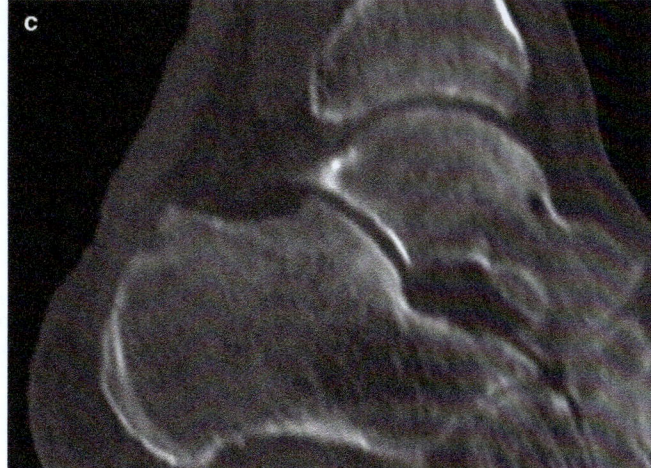

Table 5 CASPAR criteria for psoriatic arthritis

Inflammatory articular disease (joint, spine, or entheseal)
AND
At least 3 points from the following elements:
• Psoriasis: current (2 points)
Personal history (1)
Or family history (first or second degree) (1)
• Psoriatic nail distrophy (onychodystrophy) (1)
• Dactylitis: current (1)
History (diagnosed by a rheumatologist) (1)
• Negative rheumatoid factor (1)
• Radiographies (hands and feet) with juxta-articular new bone formation (excluded osteophytes) (1)

Table 6 Classification of the spondyloarthritis

	Prevalence ≈
Spondyloarthritis	0.8%
Predominant axial spondyloarthritis	
−Ankylosing spondylitis	0.3%
−Non-radiographic axial spondyloarthritis	0.2%
Peripheral spondyloarthritis	
−Associated with psoriasis: psoriatic arthritis	0.2%
−Associated with inflammatory bowel disease (Chron's/ulcerative colitis): IBD-associated arthritis	0.075% for each
−Reactive arthritis	0.01%
−Juvenile spondyloarthritis	0.01%
+/− SAPHO syndrome	0.04%

Treatment [61]:

- **NSAIDs** (+++)
- +/− **methotrexate**, leflunomide, sulfasalazine (do not have an action on the enthesitis)
- +/− biotherapies: anti-TNF-α

Evolution [76]:

- Variable:
   - Severe (20% of cases): rapidly destructive arthritis
   - Very moderate (20% of cases): absence of articular destruction

Table 7 Comparison of the two main types of spondyloarthritis

	Ankylosing spondylitis	Psoriatic arthritis
Prevalence	0.3%	0.2%
Sex	Men	M/F = 1
Age	20–30 years	30–50 years
Heredity	Yes	Yes
Axial skeleton involvement	++++ (sacroiliac/lumbar)	+ (cervical spine)
Appendicular skeleton involvement	+ (hip)	++++ (hands and feet, knees)
Clinical	Inflammatory tilting lumbago	Asymmetrical oligoarthritis/monoarthritis, of the lower limbs
Psoriasis	No	Yes
Enthesitis	+++ (calcaneus)	+++ (calcaneus)
Dactylitis	+	+++
Ankylosis	Yes	little
ESR and CRP	+/− ↗ at the time of attacks	+/− ↗ at the time of attacks
HLA	B27 (in 90% of the cases)	B27 (in 25% of the cases) B39/Cw6
Sacroiliac	++++ (bilateral sacroiliitis)	+ (asymmetrical/unilateral sacroiliitis)
Spine	Ascending evolution: lumbar spine, then thoracic, then cervical	Random evolution: cervical spine involved the most often
Lumbar spine	++++ Romanus lesion (squaring of the vertebra by erosion of the anterior corner on enthesitis) Syndesmophytes Arthritis and zygapophyseal ankylosis Ossification of the supra- and interspinous ligaments Inflammation or (stress) fracture of the complete ankylosed spine and development of pseudarthrosis (Andersson lesion)	+ Rare Romanus lesion Parasyndesmophytes
Thoracic spine	++ Idem lumbar spine and Costotransversal arthritis Costovertebral arthritis	+ Idem lumbar spine
Cervical spine	+ Erosions of the spinous processes (on enthesitis of the supraspinous ligament)	++ Subluxation C1-C2 Zygapophyseal arthritis Supraspinous ligament enthesitis Syndesmophytes
Hands and feet	+/− Subtalar osteoarthritis Ankle arthritis Medial tarsometatarsal arthritis	++++ Asymmetrical or unilateral arthritis of the MCP/MTP, PIP, and DIP Radial involvement (+)

- Period of exacerbation intersected with often prolonged remission
- Risk of erosion and ankylosis of the MTP and the toes

Discussion:

- Compared to the MRI, bone scan does not really have a role to play in diagnosing psoriatic arthritis. However, when a painful foot is being examined, the topography of the lesions found on a BS could orient the diagnosis toward psoriatic arthritis. Unlike the MRI which only explores one foot (10 min of minimum examination by carrying out three sequences of T1 axial, T2 fat sat sagittal, and coronal), the BS is a whole-body examination, and one can look for other evocative lesions, in particular on the hands and the cervical rachis.
- A study on 47 patients with recently diagnosed psoriatic arthritis showed that the BS is more sensitive than the clinical evaluation for counting the involved articulations: in 75% of patients, the clinical examination found oligo-arthritis (approximately two lesions), whereas the BS found approximately six lesions (involvement confirmed with ultrasound). The impact on chosen therapy was not evaluated [78]. Other studies using bone SPECT-CT and PET with FNA find the notion of **subclinical arthropathy** in psoriatic arthritis [79] and even in psoriasis without articular symptoms [80].
- Involvement of DIP of the hands is traditional in the event of psoriatic arthritis and of osteoarthritis, and the clinical distinction can be difficult. Involvement is predominant on the entheses and the periarticular bone in contact with the entheses in the event of psoriatic arthritis, whereas impairment relates primarily to cartilage and subchondral bone in the event of osteoarthritis. The resolution and the acquisition time required for a bone SPECT-CT (12 min, with risk of patient movements) currently do not allow for this level of distinction. In preclinical studies, the MRI (high resolution) and FNA PET (using PET dedicated to small animals) made it possible to visualize these differences and to differentiate psoriatic arthritis and osteoarthritis [79, 81].

Box 7

Articular involvement of the hands and feet predominate in psoriatic arthritis.

Box 8

Approximately 25% of patients with psoriasis will have a psoriatic arthritis, particularly in the event of nail psoriasis (onychodystrophy).

Box 9

Psoriatic arthritis: lesions of the hands and the feet [42, 61]:

- Arthritis:
  - **Asymmetrical** or unilateral
  - Concerning **MCP/MTP, PIP, and DIP**
  - DIP involvement evocative
  - Radial involvement (of all the ray) possible: MCP/MTP + PIP + DIP
- Bone proliferations on enthesitis sites:
  - Posterior or lower part of the calcaneal tuberosity, base of P1
  - Hyperostotic erosion
  - Periosteum apposition
- Bone impairment of the distal phalange and the nail:
  - Not very frequent, quasi-pathognomonic
  - Touches in particular P2 of the hallux

Box 10
Psoriatic arthritis: lesions of the axial skeleton [61]

- Sacroiliac: asymmetrical or unilateral sacroiliitis
- **Cervical spine**: often impaired
  - Subluxation C1-C2
  - Zygapophyseal arthritis
  - Enthesitis of the supraspinous ligament
  - Syndesmophytes (ossification of the edge of the intervertebral disc, with thin vertical bands connecting the vertebral corners)
- Thoracic-lumbar spine: less often impaired than with ankylosing spondylitis
  - No zygapophyseal arthritis
  - Enthesitis of the supraspinous ligament
  - Parasyndesmophytes: chunky and asymmetrically distributed syndesmophytes in zones not immobilized by zygapophyseal ankylosis (because no zygapophyseal arthritis), resulting in thicker, unilateral bony bridges, extending beyond the intervertebral disc (Fig. 14)
  - Enthesitis of the vertebral corners

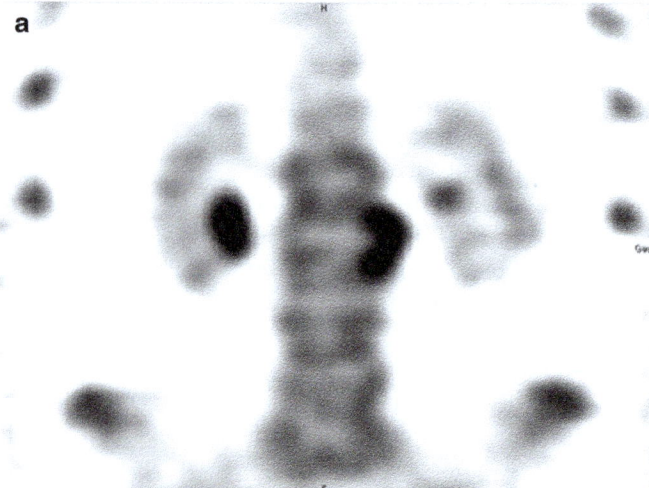
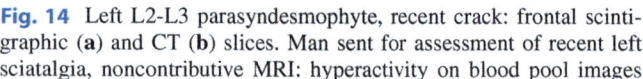
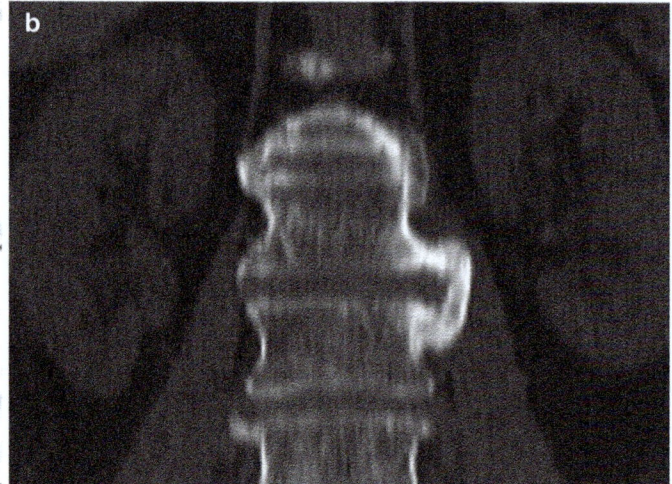

Fig. 14 Left L2-L3 parasyndesmophyte, recent crack: frontal scintigraphic (**a**) and CT (**b**) slices. Man sent for assessment of recent left sciatalgia, noncontributive MRI: hyperactivity on blood pool images (not shown) and on delayed images of the parasyndesmophyte explaining symptomatology

Diabetic Foot: Diabetic Neuropathic Osteoarthropathy (Diabetic NOA, aka Charcot Foot, Charcot Neuroarthropathy)

Predisposition [21]:

- Poorly controlled diabetes mellitus, type I or II, with peripheral neuropathy
- M/F = 1
- Average age ≈ 60 years

Past medical history: NR
Frequency:

- Rare
- Prevalence: 0.2% of the diabetics (who account for 4% of the population)

Mechanism [61, 82]:

- After several years (at least 5–10 years), the **uncontrolled hyperglycemia** impacts the feeder vessels of the peripheral nerves and is responsible for diabetic neuropathy. It is sensorimotor neuropathy, predominantly sensory, and in particular leads to reduction in the pain sensitivity. Neuropathy touches also sympathetic nerve system. The **autonomic neuropathy** leads to reduced vascular resistance and **peripheral hypervascularization**. The hypervascularization of the bone increases **bone resorption** (activation of osteoclasts) and embrittlement. In this terrain, a fracture or microfracture leads to traditional inflammatory phenomena (release of cytokines and surge of macrophages), but continued weight-bearing (unperceived nociceptive stimulus) and the preexistent hypervascularization amplify these phenomena and abruptly increase osseous resorption and the fracture risk: this **acute phase**, if it is not quickly treated (offloading), quickly leads to complications such as **multiple fractures and luxations** and leads to **definitive deformations** with the collapse of the arch of the foot.

Types: Eichenholtz classification [41, 61, 82]

- Stage I (fragmentation): acute inflammation with osseous destruction and luxation
- Stage II (coalescence): beginning of the processes of repair with bone resorption and callus formation
- Stage III (consolidation/remodeling): osseous consolidation associated almost constantly with residual deformation

Interview and clinical examination [61]:

- Stage I = **acute phase** (Fig. 15)
  - **Acute inflammation**: red, hot foot with edema, but no fever
  - Inconstant pain (sensory neuropathy)
  - No foot ulcer (= not of infectious explanation to the symptoms)
  - Palpable foot pulses, often leaping
  - Beginnving of deformation
- Stage II
  - Reduction in the acute inflammation
- Stage III = final stage (Fig. 16)
  - Foot +/− cold
  - Deformation: collapse of the arch of the foot, plantar luxation of the cuboid with overload and risks of foot ulcer

Paraclinical examination [61]:

- **Acute phase:**
  - Lab tests: WBC count, ESR, and CRP all normal
  - X-ray:
    Often normal
    Beginning of articular subluxation
  - MRI:
    Impairment predominantly on the tarsometatarsal joints and transverse tarsal joint
    Multiple bone edema of the tarsus, on both sides of joint space.
    Subchondral fracture
    Articular subluxations
    Articular effusion
- **Late stage:**
  - X-ray:
    Articular deformation
    Subchondral bone fragmentation
    Remodeling: osteosclerosis, ostephytes, etc.
    +/− lytic lesions of the MTP
  - MRI:
    Idem X-ray
    Regression of the edema

Differential:

- **Acute phase:**
  - Infection (+++)
  - Complex regional painful syndrome type I
  - Gout

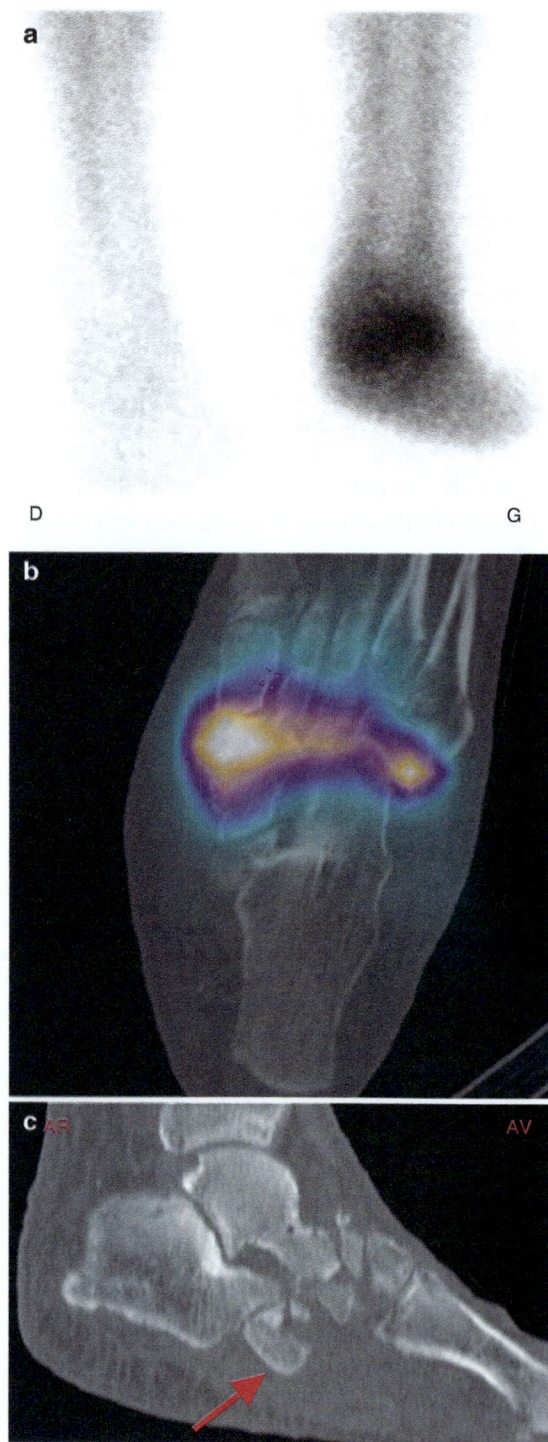

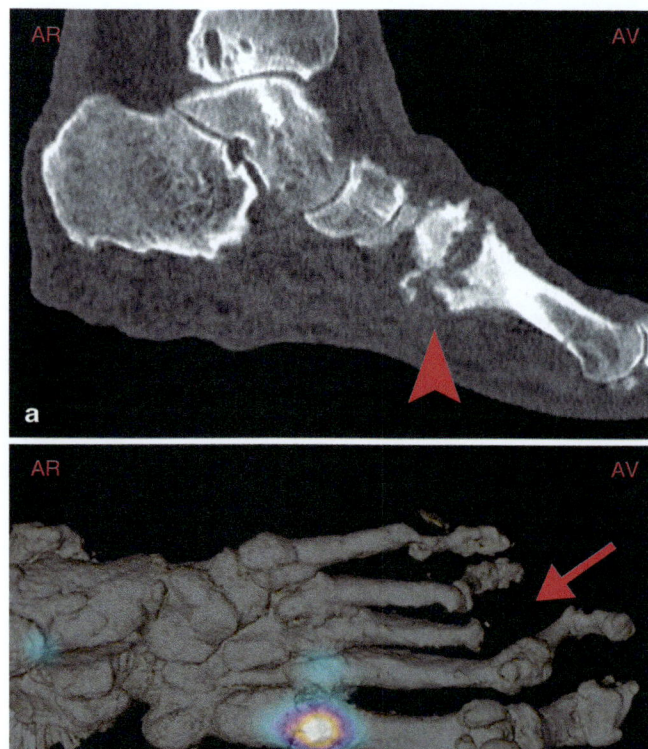

Fig. 16 A and B. Diabetic NO stage III, sagittal CT slice (**a**) and fused VRT image (**b**). Diabetic patient with known diabetic NOA of the tarsometatarsal articulation of the first ray and prior resection of the third toe (arrow). Foot ulcer on the remainder of the third ray, suspicion of osteomyelitis of the third ray: no osteomyelitis seen on the bone scan or the labeled leukocyte scintigraphy (Leukoscan, images not shown). Note moderate uptake of the diabetic NOA with joint involvement in a suggestive topography and the bone destruction at the base of M1 (arrow heads) (Images from Dr. L. Tessonnier)

- – Fracture
- – Phlebitis
- – Erysipelas

Classification: NR
Evolution:

- Acute phase:
  - – If the foot offloaded rapidly: improvement in 24–48 h
  - – If no offloading:
    Aggravation, which can be fast (in a few days)
    Multiple fractures and deformations
- Late stage:
  - – Nonphysiological weight-bearing points: foot ulcer which can be complicated by osteomyelitis, which could lead as far as amputation

Fig. 15 (**a–c**) Diabetic neuropathic osteoarthropathy stage I, front view of blood pool phase (**a**), fused transverse slice (**b**), and sagittal CT slice (**c**). 60-year-old man who has been diabetic for 20 years, with poor management and no follow-up: pain and inflammation of the left foot for the past 2 months. Aspect compatible with diabetic neuropathic osteoarthropathy on both the CT and the MRI, but there is a doubt about an superimposed osteomyelitis: bone SPECT-CT assessment. Note the polyarticular involvement of the transverse tarsal joint (telling topography), the bone destruction, and the beginning collapse of the arch of the foot with plantar luxation of the cuboid (arrow): diabetic neuropathic osteoarthopathy. No other focused bone sites and not suspicious sites on the labeled leukocyte scintigraphy (Leukoscan, images not shown): no osteitis, confirmed with patient follow-up (Images from Dr. J.B. Puech)

Treatment [41, 82]**:**

- **Acute phase:**
  - **Rapid Tx**
  - **Rest**
  - **Offloading the foot**
  - Cast/orthesis, until the local cutaneous temperature returns to normal (minimum 8 weeks)
  - +/− medication: evaluation in the course of biphosphonates, therapies targeting RANK-RANKL axis and OPG (osteoprotegerin)
- Late stage:
  - Therapeutic orthesis/shoes
  - +/− surgery depending on sequela, in order to limit the secondary risk of ulceration
- Management of diabetes

Discussion:

- Bone scans are not useful in the diagnosis of the acute or late stage of diabetic neuropathic osteoarthropathy. However, diabetic patients can have a bone scan if there is a suspicion of fracture, of infection, or of complex regional pain syndrome type I, and it is necessary to be able to mention the diagnosis of diabetic neuropathic osteoarthropathy in acute phase.

Box 11

An acute inflammation of the foot in a patient with poorly managed diabetes, without foot ulcer, must suggest diabetic neuropathic osteoarthropathy and lead to an immediate offloading and elevation of the foot.

Box 12

Diabetic NO:

  Rare pathology found in poorly managed diabetics

  Multiple and sudden fractures and luxations of the foot

  Articular involvement of the anterior tarsus in 70% of cases (Table 8)

  Risk: collapse of the arch of the foot

Table 8 Diabetic NOA: topography of lesions

Main joints concerned with diabetic NOA	
Tarsometatarsal joint	50%
Transverse tarsal joint	20%
IP and MTP joint	18%
Ankle	10%
Posterior calcaneus	2%

Diabetic Foot: Osteomyelitis

Predisposition:

- **Diabetes**
- **With foot ulcer**

Antecedents: NR
Frequency [41, 61, 83]:

- **Frequent**
- Diabetes ≈ 4% of the population
- Ulcer ≈ 20% of the diabetics
- Osteomyelitis:
  - >40% of the diabetics with ulcer
  - Responsible for >20% of hospitalizations of diabetic patients

Mechanism [41, 61]:

- After several years (at least 5 years), **uncontrolled hyperglycemia** becomes responsible for **diabetic neuropathy** and **diabetic arteriopathy**. The neuropathy is sensorimotor, predominantly sensory, and leads to **pain sensitivity disorders** and proprioception disorders, as well as a muscular atrophy which contributes to the collapse of the arch of the foot. The result is an increase from micro-injury episodes impacting the foot, which pass unperceived, and a modification of the physiological weight-bearing points. Diabetic peripheral arteriopathy is responsible for a reduction in arterial flow to the foot and for ischemia, with trophic disorders. On this weakened area, a wound can occur (1) after one or more micro-injuries and (2) on a zone of overload with hyperkeratosis subjected to shear-type force, formation of a pocket of separation under the hyperkeratosis, cracking of the hyperkeratosis, and fistulization of the pocket fluid. This **asymptomatic wound** (pain not perceived) will not heal (continued pressure and ischemia if diabetic arteriopathy) and will worsen. The **ulcer** becomes chronic and runs a high risk of infection: it progresses in depth, reaching the bone and will be responsible for an adjacent **osteomyelitis**. On this circumstance, the osteomyelitis involves a high risk of **amputation**.

Types: NR
Interview and clinical examination [61, 83]:

- **Chronic ulceration** (always! No hematogenic osteitis)
- **Two clinical presentations**:
  - Obvious infection of the soft tissues:
    Acute inflammation: red, hot foot with edema
    +/− pain
    +/− moderate fever

+/− purulent flow, collection, necrosis
  - Asymptomatic chronic ulceration apparently isolated (low-noise osteomyelitis)
- Exploration by a sterile, blunt metal probe (probe-to-bone test): **rough bone contact** (Se = 60%, Sp = 91%) [84]

Paraclinical examination [61]:

- Lab tests: ESR and CRP +/− ↗
- Bacteriology:
  - No sampling from the ulcer because:
    Colonization is near constant which is not sign of an infection
    Or germ samples are not the same as those responsible for the osteomyelitis
  - **Bone biopsy** [85, 86]:
    Gold standard, not carried out very often in practice
    Access via healthy skin, first
    Bone infection if:
      Germ isolation
      Or histological modification: inflammatory cells and osteonecrosis
- **X-ray** [86]:
  - Essential, but not very sensitive and moderately specific
  - Lesions:
    Appear tardily (>10 D)
    Cortical erosion, demineralization in the wound area
- **MRI:**
  - The most useful imaging: Se ≈ 90% and Sp ≈ 80% [84, 86]
  - Bone lesion in hypo-T1, hyper-T2 fat sat, and hyper-T1 fat sat gado
  - In the ulcer area.
- Bone scan:
  - Sensitive (≈ 85%), not very specific (≈ 30–50%) [84, 86]
  - Blood pool and delayed bone hyperactivity
  - In the ulcer area
  - Focal uptake, diffusing to the remainder of the bone
- Labeled leukocyte scintigraphy

Differential:

- Infection of the soft parts without osteomyelitis
- Diabetic NOA (Table 9)

Classification: NR
Evolution [87]:

- In spite of ATB Tx:
  - Minor amputations necessary in 60%
  - Failure/recurrence in 30%

Table 9 Diabetic foot: differential diagnosis between diabetic neuropathic osteoarthropathy (NOA) in the acute phase and osteomyelitis

Diabetic NOA in acute phase	Osteomyelitis
No foot ulcer	**Foot ulcer**
Articular	Osseous and/or articular
Polyarticular from the start	Progressive extension
Transverse tarsal and tarsometatarsal joints	In the ulcer area

Treatment [41]:

- **Preventive** Tx
- Before the ulcer:
  - Management of diabetes
  - Prevent wounds and RHD (shoes, foot care, daily self-examinations)
- At the stage of the ulcer:
  - **Emergency offloading**
  - Local care
  - +/− revascularization if necessary
  - If infection: debridement, ATB
- At the osteomyelitis stage:
  - **Emergency offloading**
  - **ATB** for 3 months
  - Or ATB for 1 month with ablation surgery of the infected bone fragment
  - +/− revascularization if necessary

Discussion:

- The diagnosis of diabetic osteomyelitis via imaging is difficult.
- The imaging available in nuclear medicine can be carried out when radiography is ambiguous and the MRI is contraindicated or not contributive.
- A bone SPECT-CT is sensitive (≈85%) but is generally little carried out because it is not very specific (≈30–50%): the FP can be diabetic neuropathic osteoarthropathy, osteoarthritis, or fracture [84, 86].
- Labeled leukocyte scintigraphy (in vitro method) has good sensitivity (≈85%) and a good specificity (≈90%) but is not readily available and more difficult to carry than MRI: it has a role to play when MRI cannot be carried out [86].
- ^{18}F-Fluorodeoxyglucose (FDG) positron emission tomography (PET) has been little studied, with series often poorly carried out (absence of gold standard) and with contradictory results. A recent meta-analysis carried out in 2013 found only nine articles of good quality. Only

Box 13
To identify or eliminate osteomyelitis is crucial for patient therapy and the prognosis of an ulcer on a diabetic foot.

Two questions, based on the clinical presentation:

- Infected ulcer: additional osteomyelitis?
- Asymptomatic ulcer: low-noise osteomyelitis?

Box 14
The diagnosis of osteitis is clinical and takes precedence over the results of imaging and bacteriology [41].

Osteomyelitis on a diabetic foot is not possible without foot ulcer.

Box 15
Diabetic foot ulcer not healed after 2 months [21, 41]:

- Offloading not strictly observed
- Underlying osteomyelitis
- Overlooked ischemia

Box 16
Diabetic foot, suspicion of:

- Diabetic NOA
- Ulcer
- Osteomyelitis
  - ATT: emergency offloading

four studies (of which two using PET without CT) representing 178 patients could be used to calculate sensitivity and specificity: Se = 74% (IC 95%: 60–85%) and Sp = 91% (IC 95%: 85–96%) [88]. In diabetic patients, the optimal conditions during the FDG injection are poorly standardized: acceptable maximum glycemia, interval between FDG injection and oral hypoglycemic agent, insulin intake, etc. [85].

Complex Regional Pain Syndrome I (CRPS I, aka Algodystrophia, Reflex Sympathetic Dystrophy Syndrome)

Predisposition [10, 89]:

- Women (ratio M/F = 1/3)
- Adults (90%) > children, teenagers (10%)
- Depression and anxiety: discussed, often associated with the CRPS I but more probably a consequence than a preexistent state

Past medical history [10, 89]:

- Recent trauma (+++), whatever its intensity (fracture, sprain, etc.)
- Surgery
- Injection, local infection, burns, frostbite, etc.
- 10% of the patients do not report any triggering event

Frequency:

- Incidence = 25 cases per 100,000 person-years

Mechanism [90, 91]:

- Precise mechanism little understood
- There are eight major concepts regarding the etiology of CRPS I:
  - Inflammatory process
  - Sympathetic nerve dysregulation
  - Autoimmune cause
  - Ischemic phenomenon
  - Sensitizing of the central nervous system
  - Lesion of the peripheral nervous system
  - Reorganization of the cerebral cortex
  - Neuronal inflammation

Types [90]:

- **Early stage (hot)**: pain, hot limb (Fig. 17)
- **Late stage (cold)**: pain, stiffness, atrophy, cold member
- Traditional evolution of the hot stage to the cold stage
- Cold stage from the start is possible, in particular in children and teenagers (Fig. 18)

Interview:

- **Pain (+++)** (absent in 5% of patients):
  - **In a limb** (sup. Limb a little more often than inf. limb)
  - Permanent
  - Disproportionate to any inciting event
  - Spontaneous and caused

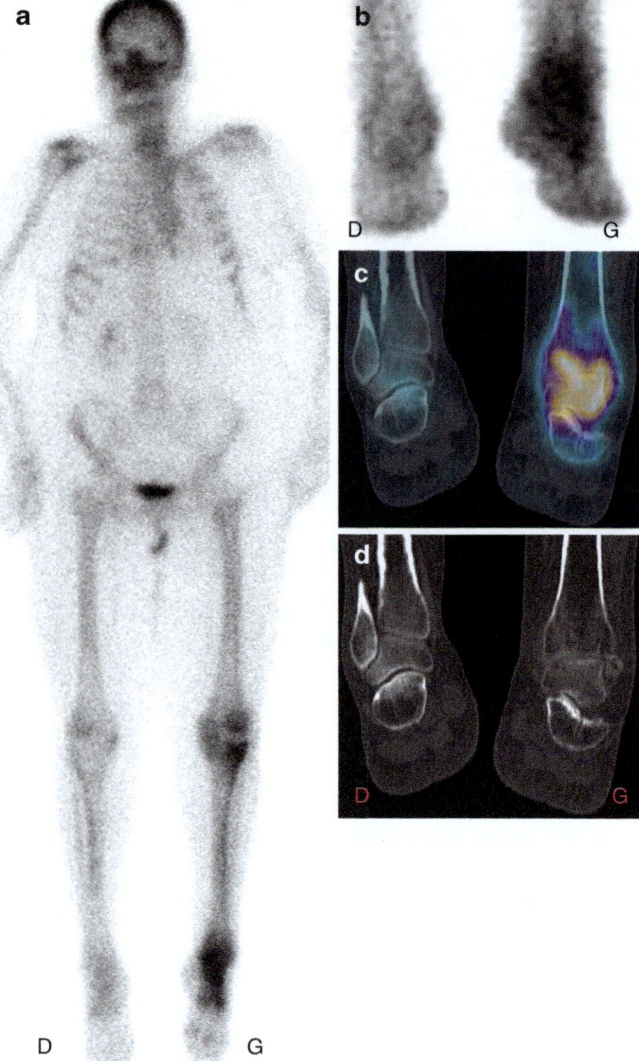

Fig. 17 CRPS I hot form of the left lower limb in an adult, front views of WB (**a**) and blood pool phase (**b**), frontal fused (**c**), and CT (**d**) slices. Trauma 5 months prior, with treated fractures of the left lateral malleolus and the proximal epiphysis of the left tibia, persistence of pain and edema. Overall hyperactivity of the left lower limb, visible also on blood pool phase (abnormal more than 3 months after the trauma)

- Burn
- Hyperalgesia
- Allodynia (painful feeling with a nonpainful stimulus)

Clinical examination:

- **Vasomotor disorders**:
  - Hot stage: heat, redness
  - Cold stage: coldness, paleness
- **Sudomotor disorders and edema**:
  - Hot stage: edema, sudation
  - Cold stage: cutaneous dryness

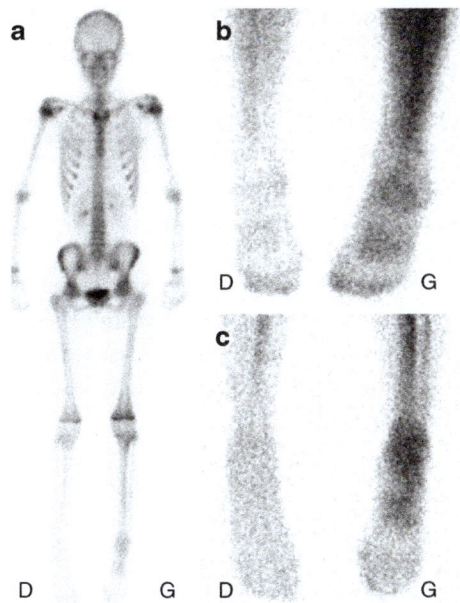

Fig. 18 CRPS I, cold stage of the right leg in a 15-year-old girl: front views of WB (**a**), blood pool (**b**), and delayed (**c**) images

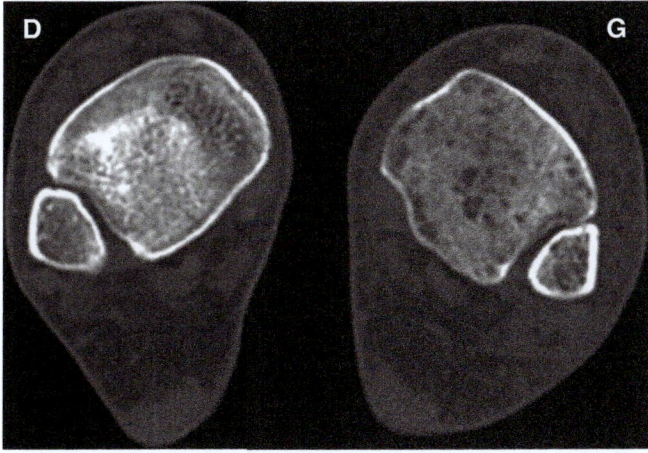

Fig. 19 Lacunar osteoporosis of the left foot on CRPS I, transverse CT slice of the ankles

- **Trophic and motor disorders**:
  - Hot stage: stiffness
  - Cold stage: stiffness, thin skin, depilation, capsulo-ligamentary retraction

Paraclinical examinations: (examinations used to eliminate differential diagnoses)

- Lab tests: no inflammatory syndrome.
- X-ray/CT:
  - Diffuse lacunar osteoporosis ("patchy") (Fig. 19)
  - Osteoporosis is not pathognomonic to CRPS I and can also be seen in the event of disuse [92]

- EMG: if carried out, normal
- Bone scan:
  - Hot stage: blood pool and delayed hyperactivity
  - Cold stage [93]:
    Following a hot stage: normal or low blood pool activity, moderate and even high delayed uptake
    From the start: blood pool and delayed hypoactivity

Differential:

- Antalgic disuse of a limb: leads to blood pool and delayed hypoactivity on the bone scan which could lead one to believe the patient has cold stage CRPS I (or even suggest hot stage CRPS I in the controlateral limb)
- CRPS II (aka: causalgia): subtype of CRPS with evidence of peripheral nerve injury
- Infections
- Neuropathy: peripheral (mononeuropathy, crushing, etc.), central, diabetic, infectious, etc.
- Vascular disorders: arterial (Raynaud syndrome, atherosclerosis) or venous (phlebitis)
- Inflammatory disease: RA, osteoarthritis, etc.
- Trauma: stress fracture, sprain

Classification:

- **Budapest clinical criteria: Se = 99%, Sp = 68%** [91, 94]
  1. Continuing pain, which is disproportionate to any inciting event
  2. Must report at least one symptom (*felt by the patient*) in three of the four following categories:
     Sensory: reports of hyperesthesia
     Vasomotor: reports of temperature asymmetry and/or skin color changes and/or skin color asymmetry
     Sudomotor/edema: reports of edema and/or sweating changes and/or sweating asymmetry
     Motor/trophic: reports of decreased range of motion and/or motor dysfunction (weakness, tremor, dystonia) and/or trophic changes (hair, nail, skin)
  3. Must display at least one sign at time of evaluation (*noted by the clinician*) in two or more of the following categories:
     Sensory: evidence of hyperalgesia (to pinprick) and/or allodynia (to light touch and/or temperature sensation and/or deep somatic pressure and/or joint movement)
     Vasomotor: evidence of temperature asymmetry (>1 °C) and/or skin color changes and/or asymmetry
     Sudomotor/edema: evidence of edema and/or sweating changes and/or sweating asymmetry

Motor/trophic: evidence of decreased range of motion and/or motor dysfunction (weakness, tremor, dystonia) and/or trophic changes (hair, nails, skin)

4. There is no other diagnosis that better explains the signs and symptoms.

- **Budapest criteria for research: SE = 70%, Sp = 79–94%** [94, 95]
  - ≈ idem clinical criteria
  - Must present at least one symptom **in all four** symptom categories and at least one sign (observed at evaluation) in two or more sign categories [94]
  - Criteria used for research purposes, ↗ Sp to reduce the FP among the sample of patients [95]

Evolution (Table 10) [91]:

- **Persistent sequelae:**
  - In 15% of patients after 6 years
  - Pain (+++), with or without vasomotor, edema and trophic disorders
  - More frequent in the event of initial cold stage (in adults)
  - More frequent in the event of absence of cure/improvement after a 1 year
- **Work stoppage:**
  - Of at least 3 months for the majority of the patients
  - Often 12 months or more
  - Inaptitude or even job loss in 10–20% of patients

Treatment [91]:

- Early care
- Four treatment approaches:
  - Information/advice/self-responsibilization
  - Physiotherapy: physical and functional rehabilitation (encouraging the patient to use the painful limb)
  - Psychotherapy/cognitive-behavioral therapy
  - To decrease the pain: drugs, interventions

Discussion:

- In a study in 82 patients with acute (≤6 months) CRPS I, included only if they had an abnormal uptake in both blood pool and delayed images on bone scan, treatment

with high levels of biphosphonates IV (neridronate) for 10 days leads to more remissions, lasting to 1 year, than a placebo [96].

- Taking the Budapest research criteria as a gold standard, a study of 116 patients in pain, of which 69 had CRPS I, showed that BS has little diagnostic value: Se = 40% and Sp = 76%. The typical three-phase increased uptake pattern has a positive predictive value of 65% (13/20), and the three-phase decreased uptake pattern has a positive predictive value of 77% (7/9). Interestingly, hypoactivity during the blood flow and blood pool phase has a positive predictive value of 86% (19/22), independently of the delayed activity [97].

Box 17
- Diagnosis of CRPS I is clinical.
- The Budapest clinical criteria allow for a CRPS I diagnosis with a good sensitivity and specificity.
- Paraclinical examinations make it possible to eliminate the differential diagnoses.

Box 18
Specific characteristics of the CRPS I in children [91]:

- Rarer (10%), touches young teenagers (8–10 years)
- Initial cold form > hot form
- Involvement of inf. Limbs more frequent (80%)
- Primarily treated by physiotherapy (+/− intensive) and cognitive and behavioral therapy
- More favorable evolution
- More relapses (≈ 40%) but favorable evolution
- Possible sequelae in adulthood: spontaneous pain or pain after effort (≈ 50%)

Table 10 Evolution of CRPS I under treatment [91]

At 1 year:	At 6 years:
− Cure = 0–5%	− Cure = 30%
− Improvement of symptoms = 80%	− Improvement of symptoms = 55%
− No improvement = 20%	− Persistent sequelae = 15%

Gout

Predisposition [61, 89]:

- **Men** (M/F $\approx$ 5)
- > 40 years old
- Diet rich in purines (meat, seafood, beer, and strong alcohol)

Antecedents:

- Genetic factors: Family antecedents of gout in 30–50% of cases

Frequency [41, 61]:

- **Frequent**
- Prevalence: 1%
- Prevalence in men over the age of 75: 7% [98]
- The most frequent cause of inflammatory arthritis in men over 40 years of age

Mechanism [61]:

- Presence of **hyperuricemia** due to excessive production of urate (food contributions +++) and/or insufficient elimination (genetic mutation responsible for a disorder of the urinary excretion +++). The hyperuricemia causes urate **crystallization** in some **joints**: local articular factors favor crystallization, in particular in the first MTP. Urate crystals detach in the synovial fluid leading to phagocytosis by articular monocytes/macrophages which suddenly secrete inflammatory mediators, responsible for **acute arthritis**. This acute onset is spontaneously resolved in a few days. The progressive accumulation of urate crystals create nodules, surrounded by inflammatory cells and osteoclasts: the **tophus**. The tophus is responsible for an increase in osteoclastogenesis and secretes mediators decreasing the osteoblastogenesis: the result is **bone destruction**. By phenomena that are less well understood, gout is also responsible for **osseous neoformation**: spikes, osteophytes, and condensation.

Types [61]:

- Acute gout or gout attack: early stage
- Chronic tophaceous gout: late stage

Interview and clinical examination:

- **Acute gout** [41, 61, 98]:
  - **Acute monoarthritis** (+/− oligoarthritis):
    Sudden, often at night
    Intense pain
    Articular tumefaction
    Impossible mobilization
    Peripheral skeleton (lower limbs +++):
      First MTP (+++, initial site in at least 50% of cases = "podagra")
      First PIP, tarsometatarsal joints
    General signs:
      +/− fever, shivers
      +/− prodromal symptoms: irritability, asthenia
- **Chronic tophaceous gout** [61]:
  - Occurs several years ($\approx$ 5 years) after the first acute gout attack, in the absence of adapted Tx.
  - **Tophus** (++++):
    Firm and white tumefaction
    Particularly touches the cartilage, the bone, and the tissues surrounding the peripheral joints [98]
    Predominantly olecranon process, prepatellar, on the dorsal surface of the fingers and toes and on the calcaneal tendon
    Can be compressive, could fistulize, etc.
  - Uric acid stone ($\approx$ 30%) and renal insufficiency
  - Association with a metabolic syndrome and cardiovascular incidents

Paraclinical examination [61]:

- **Acute stage:**
  - Lab tests:
    ESR and CRP often $\nearrow$
    Uricemia: can be normal at the time of the crisis
  - Imaging usually not necessary
  - X-rays: normal
  - Joint aspiration (+++):
    Monosodium urate crystals (+++): Sp close to 100% [99]
    No germs
    Nonessential in the event of typical acute gout attack of the first MTP [98]
- **Chronic stage:**
  - Labs: hyperuricemia
  - X-rays:

Tophus (++++):

+/− dense (crystalline deposits)

Lower limbs

Asymmetrical

Para-articular, subcutaneous, and intraosseous

Bone destruction:

Clearly defined

In contact with the tophi

Large in size

No joint narrowing

Bone proliferation:

Spikes prolonging erosion

Bulky osteophytes/enthesophytes (responsible for "roughcast foot" in profile)

Impacting:

Feet: first MTP (+++), sesamoid, other MTP, IP, tarsometatarsal, mediotarsal

Knee: femur, tibia, and patella

Hands and wrists: IP (+++), in advanced forms

– CT: more precise evaluation the osseous and articular repercussions of the tophi

Differential:

- Acute phase: septic arthritis, another microcrystalline arthritis
- Chronic stage: ≈ none (diagnosis of gout already made)

Classification [99]:

- Diagnosis is confirmed by finding monodosium urate crystals in the synovial fluid. For a trained anatomopathologist, Sp nears 100%, which is enough for clinical practice.
- When the microscopic examination of the synovial fluid is not possible, there are five clinical classifications but which all have limitations, in particular for their use in clinical research: a new ACR/EULAR classification is being prepared (work began in 2013).

Evolution [41, 61, 98]:

- **Acute stage:**
  – Spontaneously resolved in 5–10 days.
  – Resolved in 2 days under colchicine.
  – Evolution by crises several months or years apart: in the absence of Tx, a second acute attack often occurs within 2 years.

- **Chronic stage:**
  – In the absence of adapted Tx
  – A few years after the first crisis
- **Comorbidities (+++)**: HTA, diabetes, dyslipidemia, renal pathologies

Treatment [41, 61]:

- **Acute stage:**
  – Colchicine
  – +/− NSAIDs, oral corticotherapy
- **In the long term**: **to reduce the uricemia**
  – **Dietetic rules**: weight reduction, restriction of purine-rich food, reduction of alcohol, beer, and sweetened soda intake
  – Medication if necessary:
    Inhibitors: allopurinol (with colchicine in the beginning to avoid attacks)
    +/− uricosuric

Discussion:

- Bone scan is not useful in acute gout or chronic gout. Chronic phase lesions should be recognized if a foot scan is being done for another problem.

> **Box 19**
> Gout and osteoarthritis can be associated, in particular on the first MTP.

> **Box 20**
> Uricemia [98]:
> Asymptomatic hyperuricemia does not necessarily lead to the development of gout: it does not require medical Tx.
> Uricemia can be normal with the acute gout (↗ of the renal excretion during the attack).
> Uricemia is always high during the chronic stage.

Part II

Anatomy

Anatomy

Bones: Structure (Fig. 1)

Bone tissues can be divided into cortical bone (or dense bone, compact bone) and spongy bone (or trabecular bone) [50, 100].

Hard, dense **cortical bone** is composed of units called osteons (or haversian systems). Osteons are made up of several concentric lamellae, formed of bone matrix [51]. Osteons run parallel to the longitudinal axis of the bone. Space between the different osteons is filled by interstitial lamellae, remains of old osteons (continual remodeling of the bone). The internal and external circumference of the cortical bone consists of internal and external circumferential lamellae, respectively.

Spongy bone is weaker and less dense. It is composed of bony trabeculae going in different directions such as to resist mechanical load distribution as best as possible. The trabeculae delimit small cavities containing of red (hematopoietic) bone marrow. Each trabecula is friable, but the total mass of the trabeculae and the way they fit together are adapted to the lines of force making the structure very resistant.

The **periosteum** constitutes the external envelope of the bones. It is a solid fibrous membrane made up of two layers: a fibrous external layer and an osteogenic internal layer. The periosteum is where the tendons and the ligaments attach to the bone. The periosteum covers the totality of the bone, with the exception of the articular cartilage. The periosteum contributes to innervation, growth, and bone healing [53].

The **endosteum** constitutes the internal envelope of the bones and resembles the periosteum. It lines the medullary cavity and the trabeculae of the spongy bone.

The **medullary cavity** constitutes the central part of the diaphysis in long bones. The medullary cavity contains vessels, nerves, and yellow bone marrow (with fat).

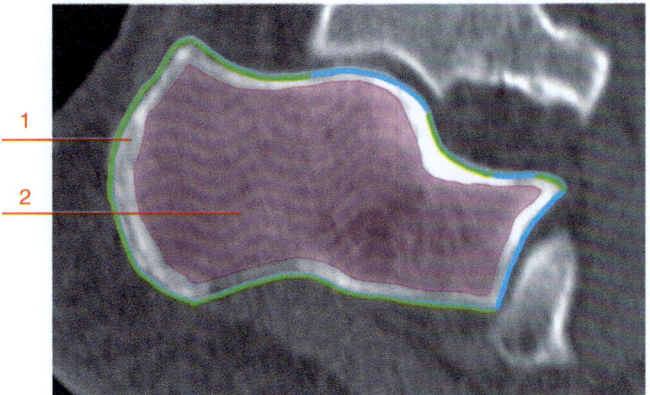

Fig. 1 Structure of a short bone. Calcaneus, sagittal CT slice. In pink: red bone marrow between the bone trabeculae. In blue: articular cartilage. In green: periosteum. NB: The endosteum is not represented on this diagram. (1) Cortical bone. (2) Spongy bone

Bones: Shape (Fig. 2)

Based on their appearance, bones can be classified into long bones, short bones, flat bones, and other varieties (irregular, pneumatic, etc.). The ankle and the foot contain only long bones and short bones.

Short bones (e.g., the calcaneus) are made of spongy bone covered with a thin layer of cortical bone.

Long bones (e.g., the tibia) are composed of proximal and distal epiphyses and a central diaphysis. The metaphysis is the junction between the diaphysis and the epiphysis [51]. The epiphyses are made of spongy bone, covered with a thin layer of cortical bone. The diaphysis is made up of a thick cylinder of cortical bone around a medullary cavity.

Fig. 2 (**a–c**) Structure of a long bone. Lower end of the tibia, frontal CT slice (**a**). Diaphysis of the tibia, transverse CT slice (**b**). Composition of the cortical bone, transverse slice (**c**, based on image by Dr. N. Macagno). In pink: red bone marrow between trabeculae. In yellow: yellow bone marrow in the medullary cavity. In blue: articular cartilage. In green: periosteum. In dark green: endosteum. NB: The endosteum is not represented on diagram (**a**). (1) Medullary cavity. (2) Cortical bone. (3) Spongy bone. (4) Int. circumferential lamellae. (5) Osteon. (6) Interstitial lamellae. (7) Ext. circumferential lamellae

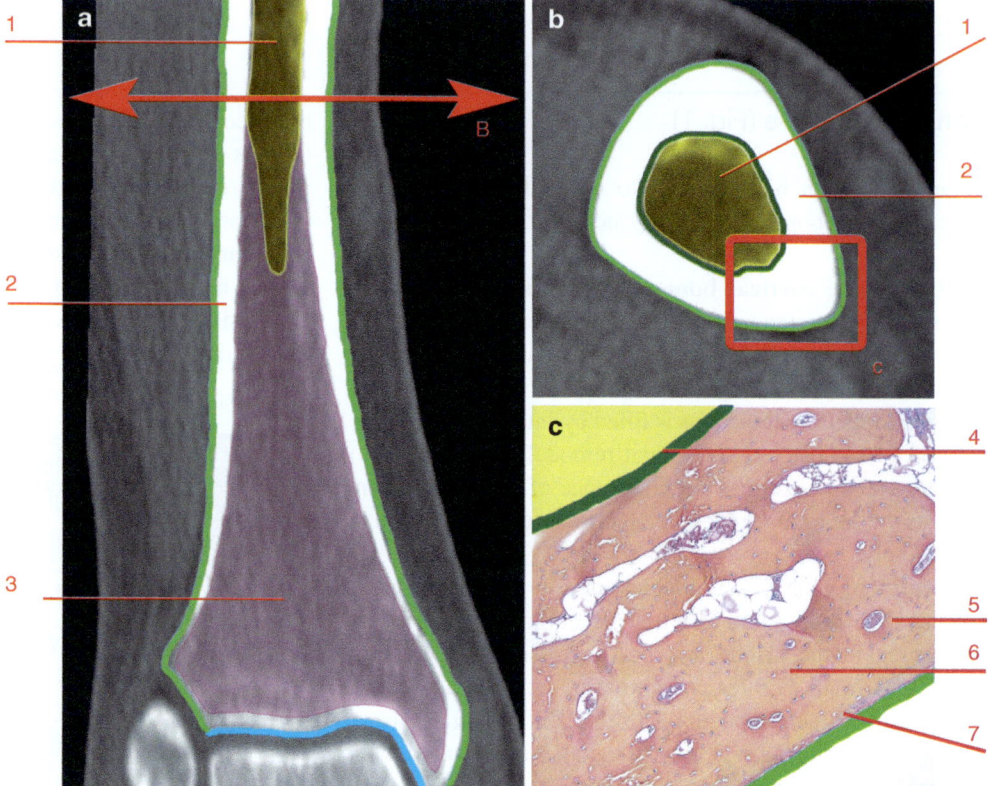

Bones: Formation (Fig. 3)

We will only provide a simplified description of long bone formation: for more details, refer to [101].

In embryos, future long bones are formed by cartilage, made up of cells (chondrocytes) in a hydrated and flexible matrix. The deformable nature of cartilage accounts for its fast growth, by division and growth of chondrocytes which secrete more and more cartilaginous matrix.

At the end of the embryonic period, the primary ossification center appears, in the middle of what will be the diaphysis. Bone progressively replaces the cartilage. The bone consists of cells (osteoblasts and osteoclasts) in a dense and rigid matrix. The osteoclasts reabsorb the cartilaginous matrix, and in space created, the osteoblasts deposit concentric layers of bone matrix.

After the birth, primarily, the secondary ossification centers appear in the epiphyses or on the periphery of the bones. In these places, the bone matrix will also gradually replace the cartilaginous matrix. The continuous elongation of the bone is ensured by the cartilage found between the primary ossification center and each secondary ossification center: the epiphyseal plate (or growth plate). As new cartilage is formed, the old is replaced by bone. The growth plate represents the bone's metaphysis, the zone of growth of the diaphysis toward the epiphysis [100].

At the end of puberty, all the epiphyseal plate has been ossified and there is no more bone growth. The place where the former epiphyseal plate was is visible on bone X-rays or scans: the epiphyseal line. The only cartilage remaining in adult bones is at the end of each epiphysis and constitutes the articular cartilage.

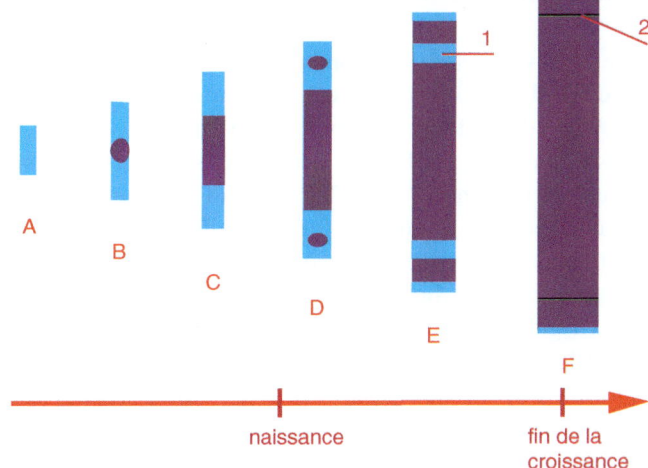

naissance

fin de la croissance

Fig. 3 Growth in length of a long bone, simplified diagram (perichondrium and periosteum not represented). In blue: cartilaginous matrix. In purple: bone matrix. (1) Epiphyseal plate. (2) Epiphyseal line. (A) Initial cartilaginous matrix. (B) Appearance of a primary ossification center in the middle of what will become the diaphysis. (C) Continuation of cartilage growth and replacement of old cartilage by bone starting at the primary ossification center. (D) Appearance of the secondary ossification centers at the level of the epiphyses. (E) Continued growth via the epiphyseal plate and replacement of the old cartilage by bone starting from the primary and secondary ossification centers. (F) End of growth. The epiphyseal plate is ossified (epiphyseal line). The only remaining cartilage is the articular cartilage at the end of the two epiphyses

Bones: Remodeling

Bone is a living tissue, constantly remodeled by **osteoclasts** and **osteoblasts**: osteoclasts reabsorb the old bone and the osteoblasts deposit new bone matrix [101, 102].

Osteoclasts (of the family of monocytes—macrophages) dig tunnels in compact bone. The walls of these tunnels are then covered with osteoblasts (of the family of fibroblasts), which secrete concentric layers of osteoid material, uncalcified bone matrix which is quickly transformed into bone matrix rigidified by calcium phosphate deposits. The concentric layers end up filling the tunnel, and the osteoblasts imprisoned in the new bone matrix are called osteocytes. Although less biologically active than osteoblasts, the osteocytes are organized in a network within the bone and will continue to take part in bone remodeling by developing or resorbing bone tissue.

The joint action of osteoclasts and osteoblasts is controlled by various protein and hormonal secretions, in particular parathormone and vitamin D, making it possible to obtain a balance between resorption and bone formation. An imbalance toward an excess of resorption leads to osteoporosis, and an excess of formation leads to osteopetrosis.

The constraints imposed on bones by gravity and muscular force guide bone remodeling, in order to adjust the bone structure to the weight bearing imposed on it. In the event of too large or inhabitual repeated constraints, bone remodeling is unbalanced toward an excess of resorption, weakening bones and possibly leading to stress fracture.

In the event of trauma involving a fracture, the bone is rebuilt quickly. The fracture site is filled by a blood clot. Stem cells in the blood clot differentiate into fibroblasts and then chondroblasts (**to the fifth day**) to create a cartilaginous callus initially linking the two edges of the fracture (**to the 20th day**). The cartilaginous callus gradually is reabsorbed and replaced by bone callus, recreating solid bone (**to 40th day**). The absence of consolidation 6–9 months after a fracture is called pseudarthrosis.

Ossification Centers of the Ankle
(Figs. 4 and 5)

The tibia presents a primary ossification center for the diaphysis and three secondary ossification centers for the tibial tuberosity, the proximal epiphysis, and the distal epiphysis.

The fibula presents a primary ossification center for the diaphysis and two secondary ossification centers for the proximal epiphysis and the distal epiphyseal.

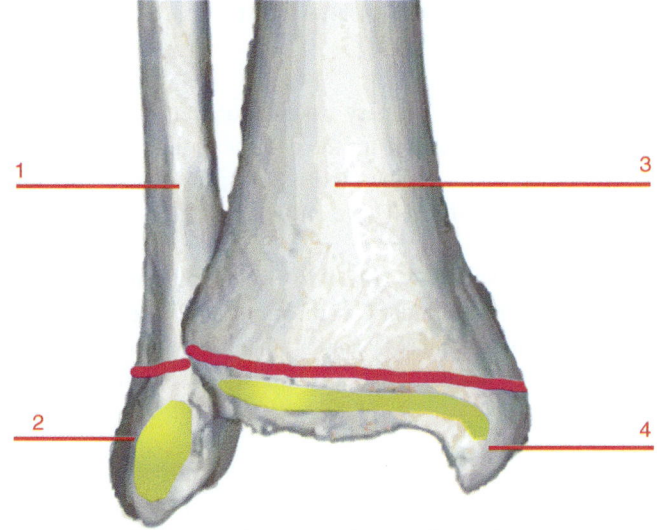

Fig. 4 Primary and secondary ossification centers of the ankle, anterior view. In yellow: secondary ossification center. In pink: epiphyseal line. (1) Fibula. (2) Lateral malleolus. (3) Tibia. (4) Med. malleolus

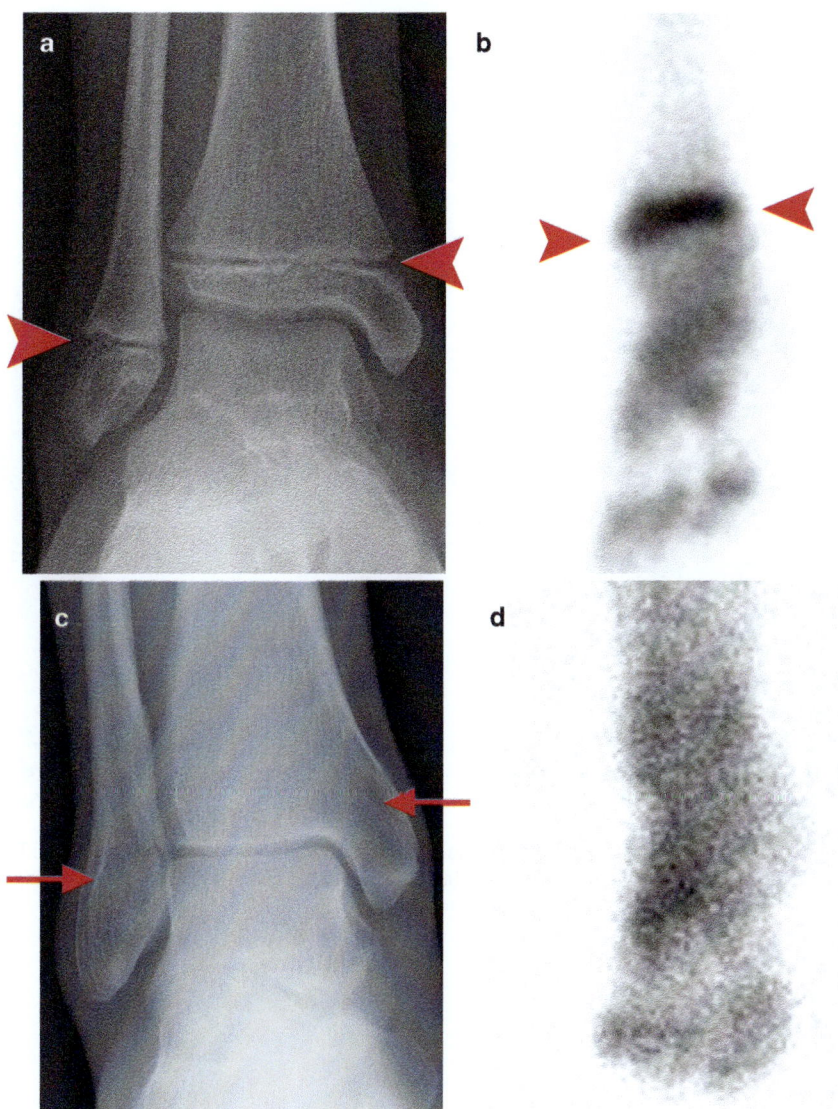

Fig. 5 (**a–d**) Ankle, epiphyseal plate, and epiphyseal lines, ant. view: normal aspect in child (**a, b**) and adult (**c, d**). Radiographic (**a, c**) and delayed scintigraphic imaging (**b, d**). Arrow head: epiphyseal plate. Arrow: epiphyseal line

Ossification Centers of the Foot
(Figs. 6 and 7)

The calcaneus has a primary ossification center and a secondary ossification center for the calcaneal tuberosity.

The other bones of the tarsus (talus, navicular, cuboid, and the three cuneiforms) have only one primary ossification center.

The metatarsals II–V (M2–M5) have a primary ossification center and a secondary ossification center for the head.

The first metatarsal (M1) and all the phalanges have a primary ossification center and a secondary ossification center for the base.

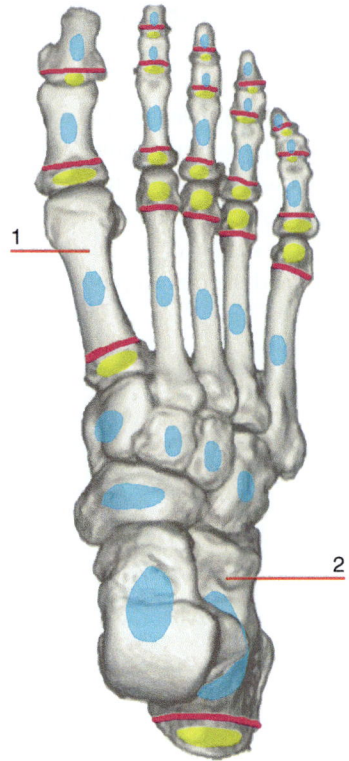

Fig. 6 Primary and secondary ossification centers of the foot, dorsal view. Diagram based on Kamina. In blue: primary ossification center. In yellow: secondary ossification center. In pink: epiphyseal line. (1) M1. (2) Calcaneus

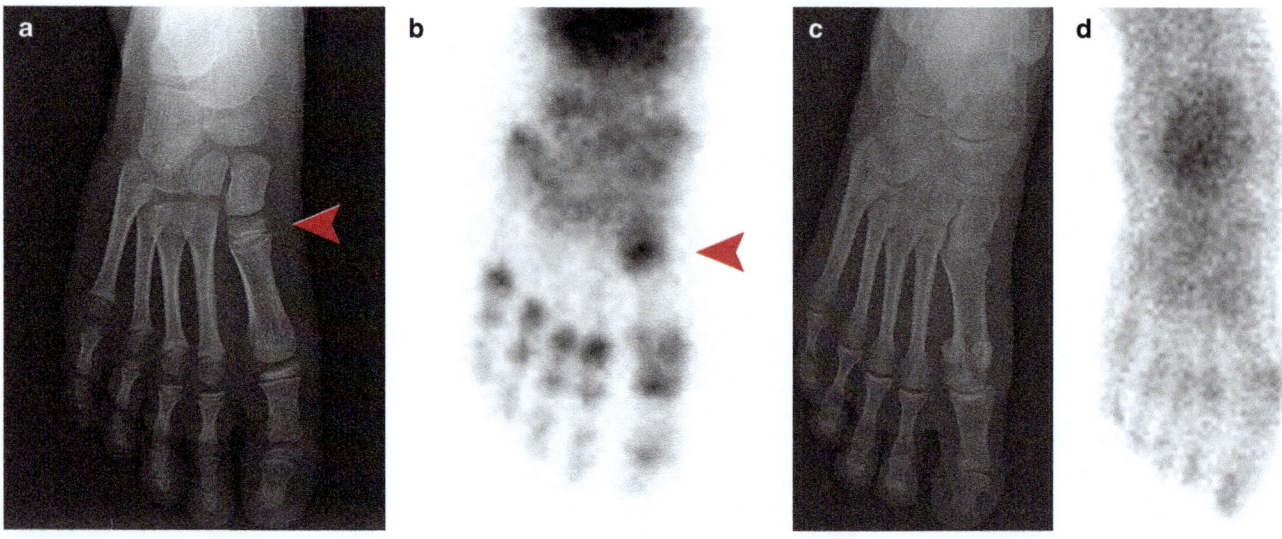

Fig. 7 (**a–d**) Foot, epiphyseal plate, and epiphyseal line, plantar view: normal aspect in child (**a, b**) and adult (**c, d**). Radiographic (**a, c**) and delayed scintigraphic imaging (**b, d**). Arrow head: epiphyseal plate of the base of M1. NB: Because of the small size of the images, not all of the epiphyseal cartilage was pinpointed by arrows

Synovial Joint: General Information
(Figs. 8 and 9)

We will again refer to Kamina's classification [51].

One distinguishes fibrous articulations (motionless), cartilaginous articulations (not very mobile), and synovial articulations (very mobile). We will develop on synovial articulations.

A synovial articulation is made up of articular surfaces, an articular cavity and an articular capsule.

The **articular surfaces** are covered with hyaline cartilage. The **articular cartilage** is avascular and is nourished primarily by imbibition via the synovial membrane, with nutritive contributions from the subjacent spongy bone [12]. The spongy bone under the articular cartilage is called **subchondral bone**.

The **articular cavity** contains the **synovial fluid**, a viscous fluid that absorbs shocks.

The **articular capsule** is made up of two membranes: **a fibrous** and very resistant membrane, in the prolongation of the periosteum and ensuring the mechanical protection of the articulation, and a **synovial membrane**, which is thin, on the deep surface of the fibrous membrane and covering the entire articulation except for the articular cartilage. The synovial membrane secretes synovial fluid and ensures the defense of the articulation against the germs.

The more mobile the articulation is, the farther from the articular cartilage the articular capsule inserts.

Inside the articulation, there can be fibrocartilaginous structures increasing congruence of articular surfaces. They are distinguished by their form: the labrum (or articular pad), the meniscus, and the articular disc. These structures are always attached to the inner side of the fibrous membrane of the articular capsule.

Joint stability is ensured by the fibrous membrane of the articular capsule, the periarticular muscular tendons, and the ligaments. These ligaments can be intracapsular (surrounded by a synovial membrane), capsular (thickening of the fibrous membrane), and extracapsular.

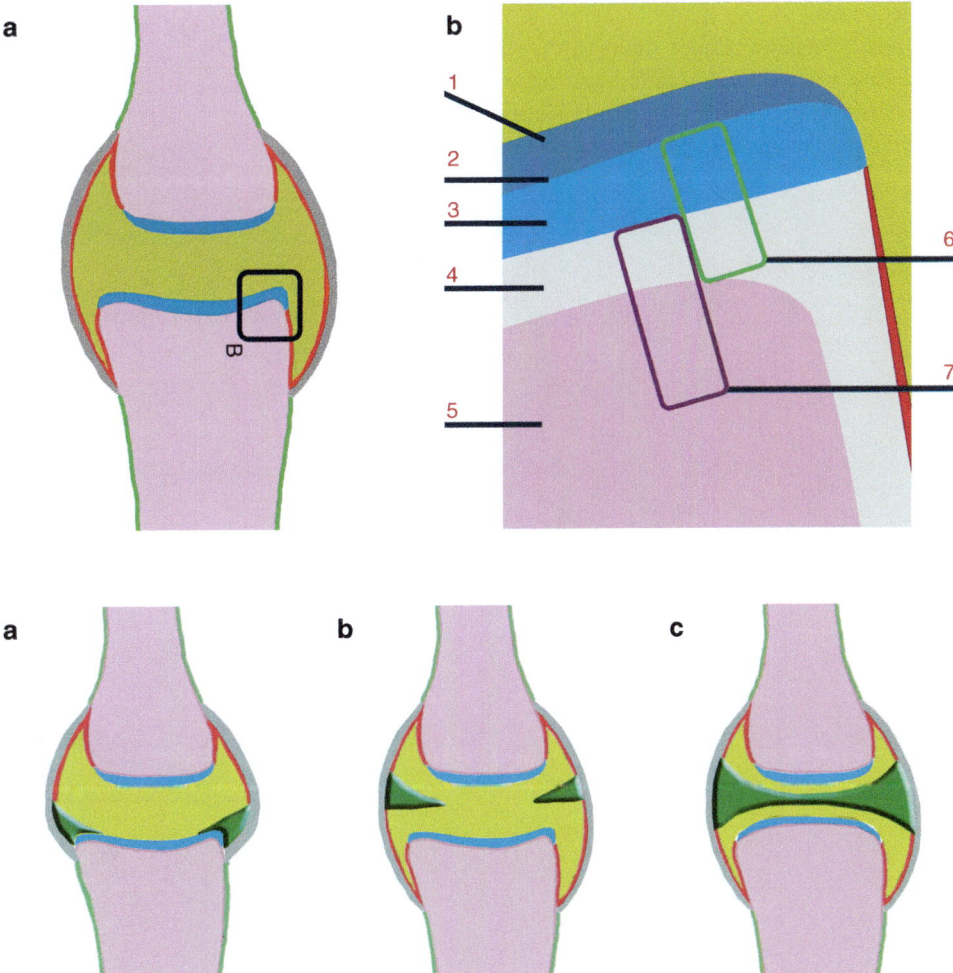

Fig. 8 (**a, b**) Synovial joint (**a**) and diagram of the subchondral bone (**b**, based on Cotten), frontal slice. In green: periosteum. In pink: spongy bone. In blue: articular cartilage. In yellow: synovial fluid. In red: synovial membrane of the articular capsule. In gray: fibrous membrane of the articular capsule.
(1) Uncalcified cartilage.
(2) Tidemark. (3) Calcified cartilage. (4) Cortical bone.
(5) Spongy bone.
(6) Osteochondral plate.
(7) Subchondral bone

Fig. 9 (**a–c**) Labrum (**a**), meniscus (**b**), and articular disc (**c**)

Tendons and Aponeuroses
(Figs. 10, 11, and 12)

Muscles can attach to bones directly with muscle fiber, via a narrow fibrous band (tendon), or a wide fibrous band (aponeurosis) [50, 51].

A **tendon** connects a muscle to a bone (NB: a ligament connects a bone to another bone). Tendons are composed of thick fibers of collagen, distributed in primarily parallel arrays following the muscle's lines of force. Tendon cells are found between the arrays—these are fibroblasts that constitute the tendon matrix.

Aponeuroses are made up of collagenous fibers, distributed around the muscle and projecting prolongations (septa) deep into the muscle to form intramuscular partitions.

A **tendon** can be divided into **three parts**: the body, the myotendinous junction, and the bone insertion (enthesis). This division has clinical importance [47].

– Myotendinous junction: the collagen fibers of the tendon spread out and fuse with collagen fibers from the muscle's aponeurosis.
– Enthesis: certain collagen fibers of the tendon spread out and fuse with the periosteum, and other collagen fibers are perforating (formerly known as Sharpey fibers), crossing the periosteum and penetrating the bone tissue.

Before its insertion on the bone, the tendon can be maintained by various fibrous structures:

– Retinaculum: a broad fibrous band stretched between two bones, maintaining the tendons
– Trochlea: small fibrous arcuate band connected to a bone, surrounding one or more tendons and serving as a pulley

In these support zones, the tendon is surrounded and protected by a synovial sheath, which allows the tendon to slip. Like the peritoneum and the pleura, the synovial sheath is a virtual serous cavity in which the tendon is invaginated.

The tendon can also be protected by a synovial bursa, which fits between the tendon and the hard bone surface.

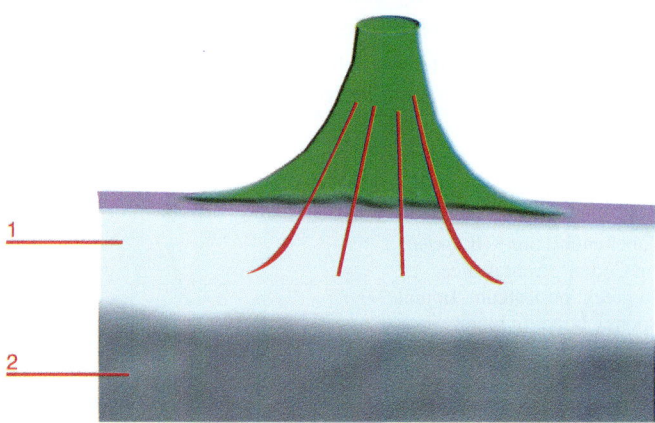

Fig. 11 Enthesis, based on Kamina. In green: tendon. In red: perforating fibers. In purple: periosteum. (1) Cortical bone. (2) Spongy bone

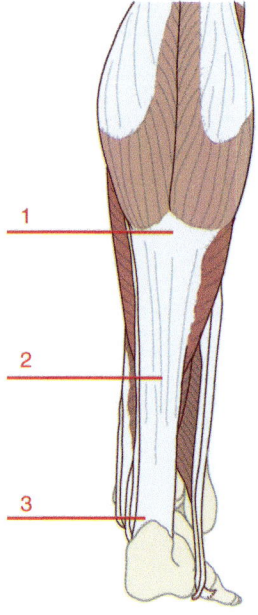

Fig. 10 Tendon, three parts: leg, posterior view. (1) Myotendinous junction. (2) Body. (3) Enthesis

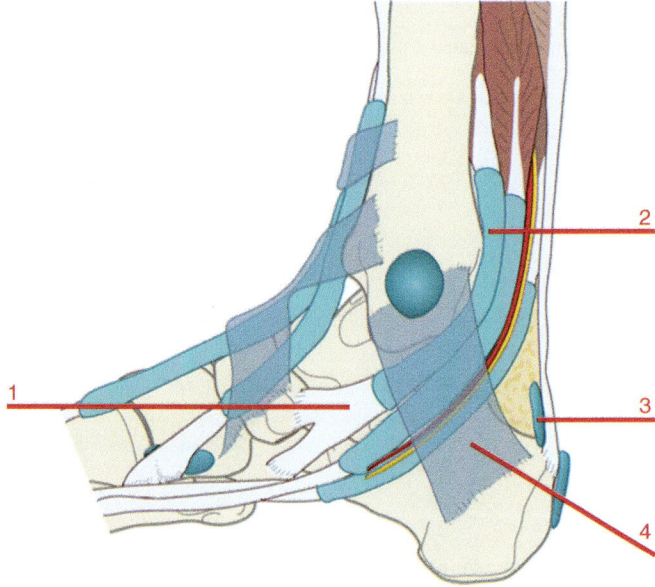

Fig. 12 Synovial sheaths and retinaculum: foot, medial view. (1) Tendon. (2) Synovial sheath. (3) Bursa. (4) Retinaculum

Ankle and Foot: General Information
(Figs. 13, 14, and 15)

The **ankle** is composed of the distal tibial epiphysis and of the distal fibular epiphysis, which form a mortise in which the talus trochlea fits.

The **foot** has 26 bones distributed from back to front in the tarsus, metatarsus, and phalanges [51].

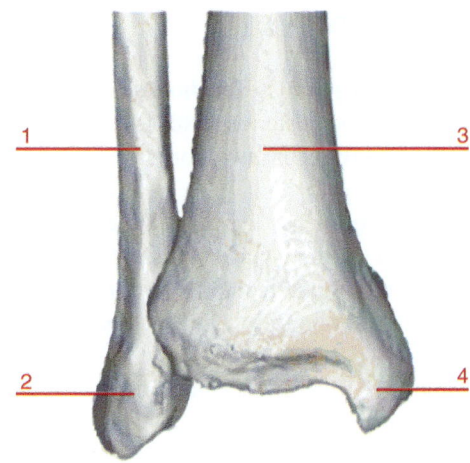

Fig. 13 Tibiofibular mortise, anterior view. (1) Fibula. (2) Lateral malleolus. (3) Tibia. (4) Medial malleolus

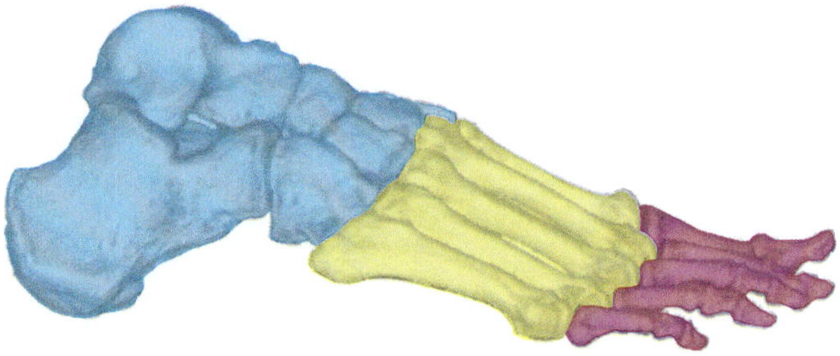

Fig. 14 The three foot bone groups, lateral view. In blue: tarsus. In yellow: metatarsus. In pink: phalanges

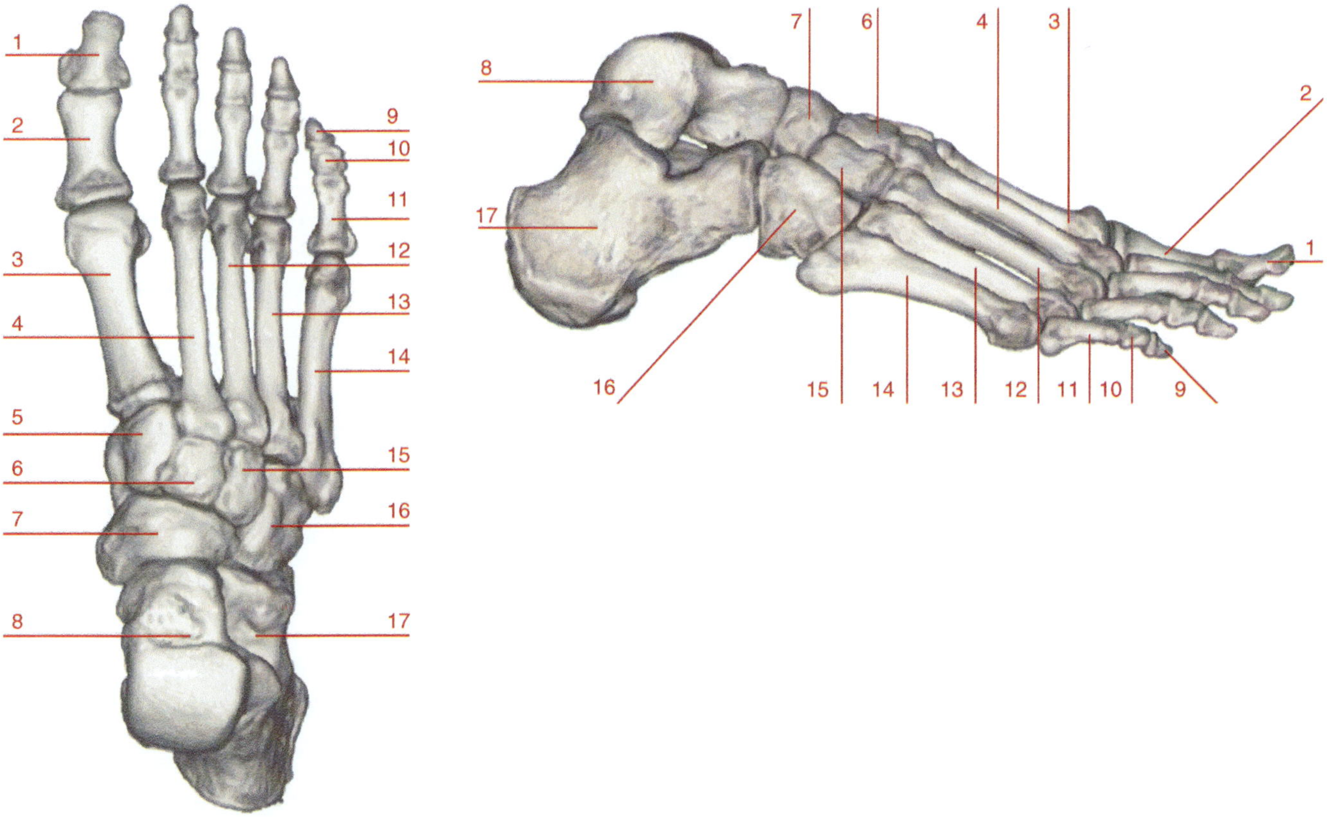

Fig. 15 (**a, b**) Foot bones, dorsal (**a**) and lateral (**b**) view. (1) Distal phalanx of the hallux. (2) Proximal phalanx of the hallux. (3) First metatarsal. (4) Second metatarsal. (5) Medial cuneiform. (6) Intermediate cuneiform. (7) Navicular. (8) Talus. (9) Distal phalanx of the fifth toe. (10) Middle phalanx of the fifth toe. (11) Proximal phalanx of the fifth toe. (12) Third metatarsal. (13) Fourth metatarsal. (14) Fifth metatarsal. (15) Lateral cuneiform. (16) Cuboid. (17) Calcaneus

Tarsus (Figs. 16 and 17)

The tarsus is composed of **seven bones**, separated into the anterior tarsus and the posterior tarsus [51, 100].

The **posterior tarsus** has two bones: the talus, above the calcaneus.

The **anterior tarsus** has five bones: the cuboid laterally, the navicular, and the three cuneiforms medially.

The anterior tarsus and the posterior tarsus are linked by the transverse tarsal joint (also Chopart joint):

– The cuboid is in front of the calcaneus.
– The navicular is in front of the talus and behind the three cuneiforms.

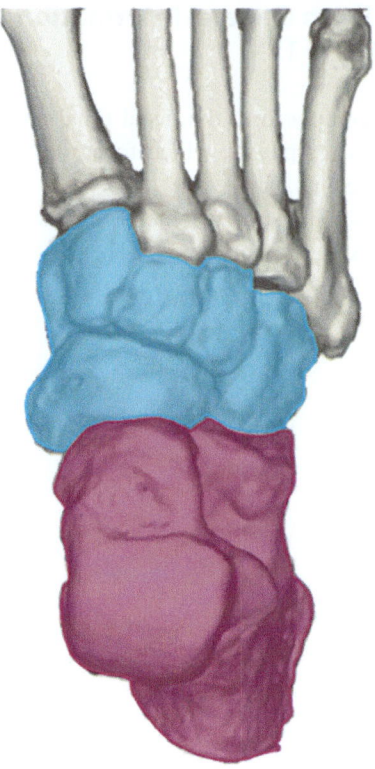

Fig. 16 Anterior tarsus and posterior tarsus, dorsal view. In pink: posterior tarsus. In blue: anterior tarsus

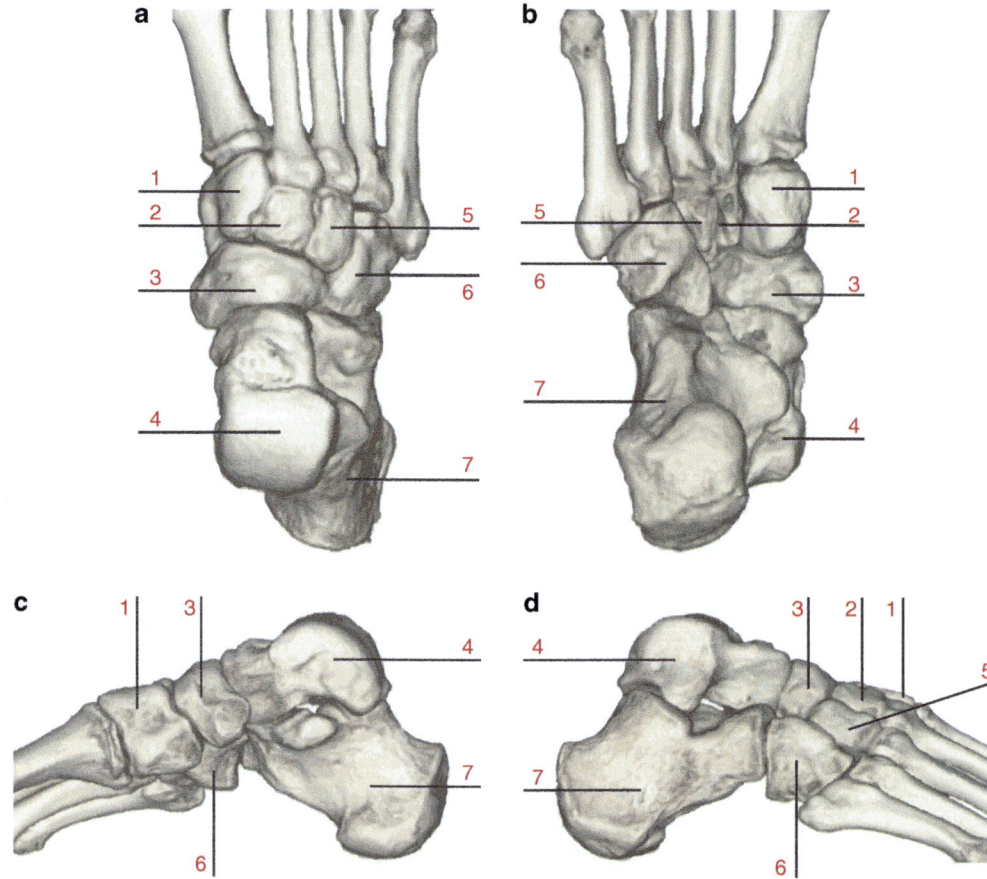

Fig. 17 Tarsus bone, dorsal (**a**), plantar (**b**), medial (**c**), and lateral (**d**) views.
(1) Medial cuneiform.
(2) Intermediate cuneiform.
(3) Navicular. (4) Talus.
(5) Lateral cuneiform.
(6) Cuboid. (7) Calcaneus

Talus (Figs. 18 and 19)

The talus is a short and dense bone, inserted in the tibiofibular mortise and transmitting the weight of the body to the calcaneus below and the navicular ahead [21]. It is a hinge bone [51]: articular surfaces account for 60% of the surface of the talus [50] (Fig. 20).

From back in front, the talus is made up of a body, a neck, and a head.

The **body of the talus** represents three quarters of the bone [51]. It presents:

- A bulky dorsal outgrowth
- A lateral process
- A posterior process

The bulky dorsal outgrowth is articulated with the tibiofibular mortise: The dorsal side or trochlea is articulated with the inferior articular surface of the tibia, the lateral surface is articulated with the lateral malleolus, and the medial surface is articulated with the medial malleolus.

The posterior process of the talus presents two tubercles—medial and lateral. Immediately behind of the lateral tubercle, there can be an accessory ossicle: the os trigonum. The fusion of the two bones gives an elongated lateral process of the talus (previously: Stieda process).

The **neck of the talus** is a narrowed portion; its plantar surface presents a deep groove, the sulcus tali.

The **head of the talus** is primarily articular and has three articular surfaces in continuity [51]:

- In the front, the navicular articular surface
- Small anterior and middle calcaneal articular facet on the plantar surface

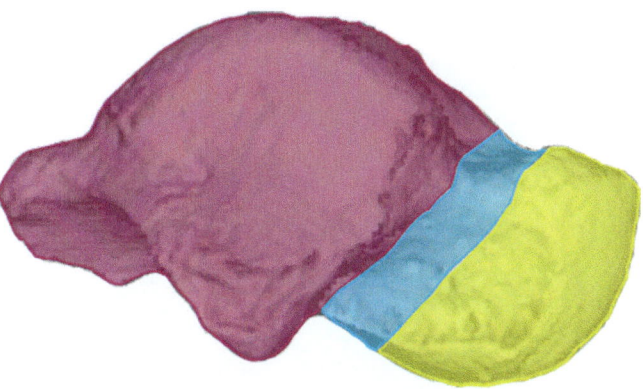

Fig. 18 Talus: three parts, lateral view. In pink: body. In blue: neck. In yellow: head

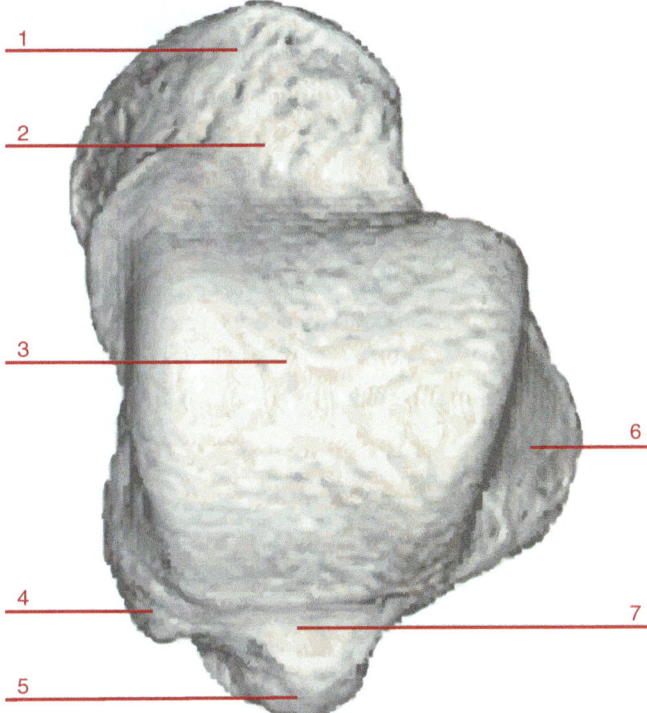

Fig. 19 Talus, posterior view. (1) Head. (2) Neck. (3) Body. (4) Medial tubercle. (5) Lateral tubercle. (6) Lateral process. (7) Posterior process

a **b**

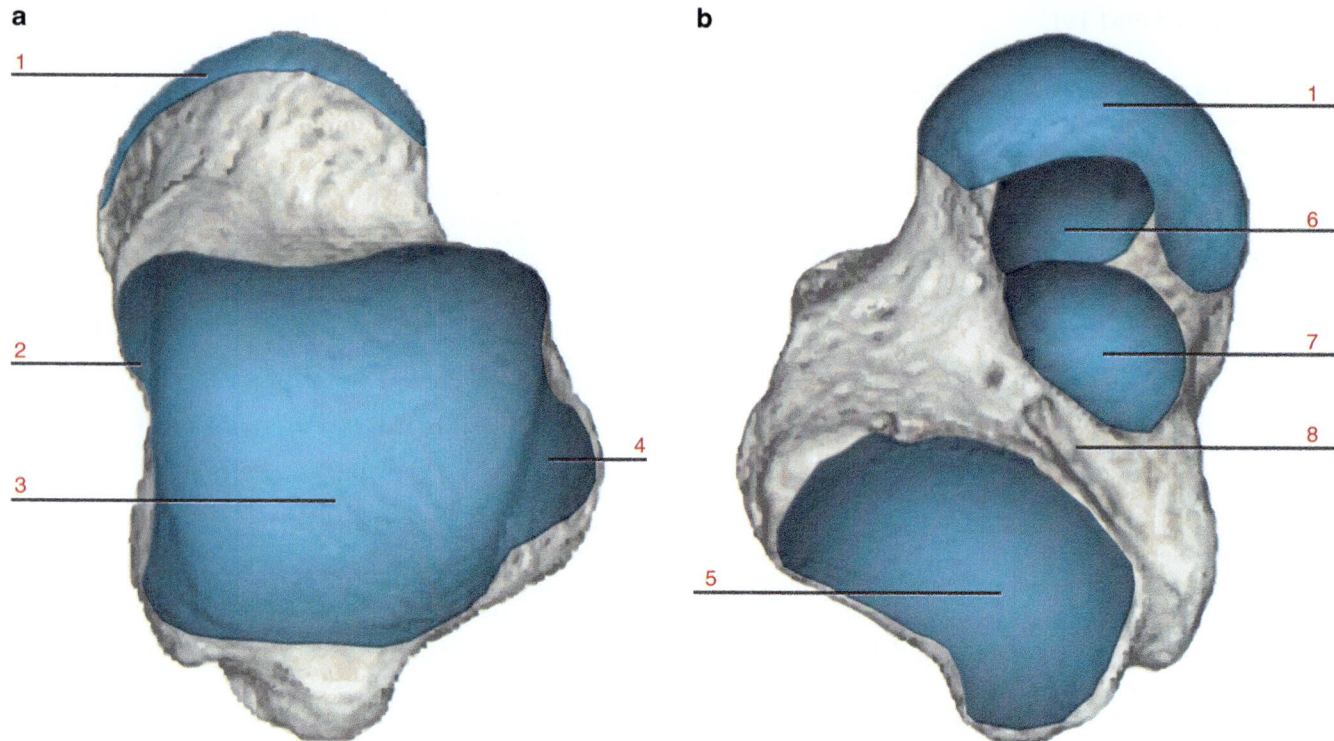

Fig. 20 (**a**, **b**) Articular surfaces of the talus, dorsal view (**a**) and plantar view (**b**). (1) Navicular articular surface. (2) Medial malleolar facet. (3) Talus trochlea. (4) Lateral malleolar facet. (5) Post. calcaneal articular facet. (6) Ant. calcaneal articular facet. (7) Middle calcaneal articular facet. (8) Sulcus tali

Calcaneus (Fig. 21)

The calcaneus is the bulkiest bone of the foot. It is located at the lower and posterior part of the tarsus and forms the projection of the heel [103]. It forms a rough rectangle and presents six surfaces.

The anterior half of its dorsal surface supports the talus and has three talar articular surfaces—anterior, middle, and posterior (the largest). The middle and posterior talar articular surfaces are separated by a groove—the sulcus calcanei, which corresponds to the sulcus tali, forming the sinus tarsi (Fig. 22).

The anterior part of the calcaneus is a little narrowed and is called the **anterior process** of the calcaneus. The anterior side is entirely articular: the cuboid articular surface. The dorsal part of the anterior process is where the bifurcate ligament inserts [51].

The lower side presents a calcaneal tubercle in the front, and the **calcaneal tuberosity** behind, where the plantar aponeurosis inserts.

The calcaneal tendon inserts in the middle of the posterior side.

The medial side has a prolongation on the upper front: the **sustentaculum tali**. The sustentaculum tali supports most of the talus [100] and is located under the middle talar articular surface [51, 103].

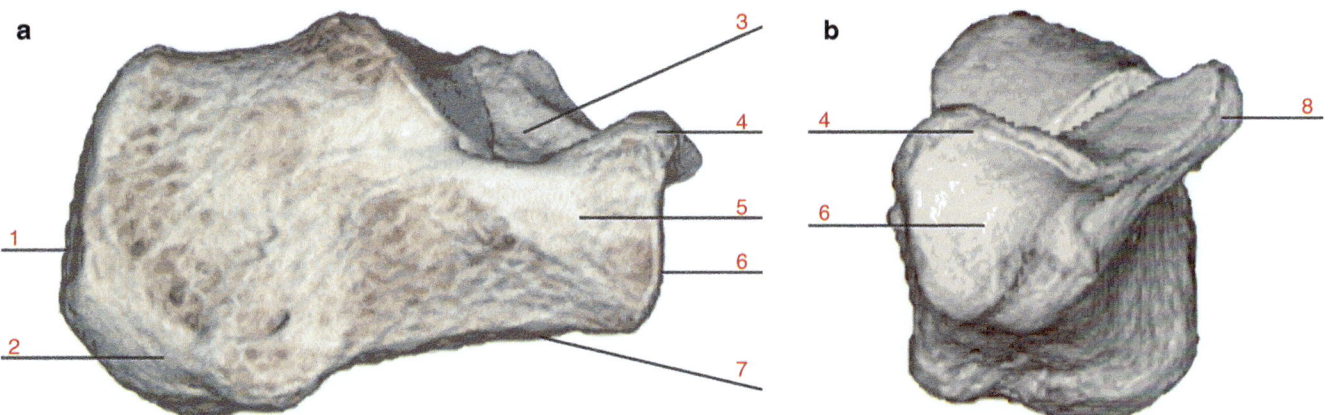

Fig. 21 (**a, b**) Calcaneus, lateral (**a**) and anterior (**b**) view. (1) Posterior surface and calcaneal tendon insertion. (2) Calcaneal tuberosity. (3) Sulcus calcanei. (4) Bifurcate ligament insertion. (5) Anterior process. (6) Ant. side. (7) Calcaneal tubercle. (8) Sustentaculum tali

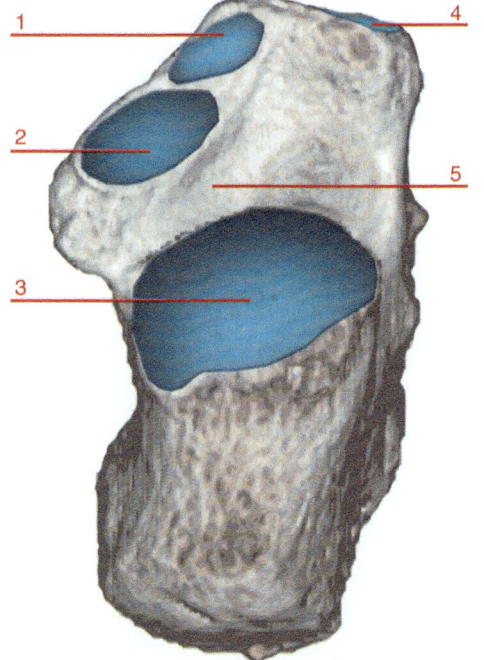

Fig. 22 Articular surfaces of the calcaneus, dorsal view. (1) Ant. talar articular surface. (2) Middle talar articular surface. (3) Post. talar articular surface. (4) Cuboid articular surface. (5) Sulcus calcanei

Anterior Tarsus: Navicular, Cuboid, and Cuneiform (Fig. 23)

The **navicular** has the shape of nacelle, lengthened from the inside out [103]. It articulates with the talus in the back and the three cuneiform in the front. Its lateral extremity articulates with the cuboid. Its medial end is palpable and forms the **tuberosity of navicular** on which the primary end of the tibialis posterior tendon inserts. Immediately behind the tuberosity, there can be an accessory bone: the accessory navicular.

The **cuboid** articulates with the calcaneus behind, the fourth and fifth metatarsals in the front, and the navicular and the lateral cuneiform medially. In the back, its plantar surface presents a prolongation under the calcaneus: the **calcaneal process**, which supports the calcaneus [51, 100]. In the middle of the plantar surface is the tuberosity of cuboid.

The **cuneiform bones** are **three** in number: medial, intermediate, and lateral; they all articulate with the navicular in the back. The medial cuneiform articulates in the front with the first metatarsal and laterally with the intermediate cuneiform and the second metatarsal. The intermediate cuneiform articulates in the front with the second metatarsal, in the middle with the medial cuneiform and laterally with the lateral cuneiform. The lateral cuneiform bone articulates in the front with the third metatarsal, in the middle with the intermediate cuneiform and the second metatarsal, and laterally with the cuboid and a small part with the fourth metatarsal.

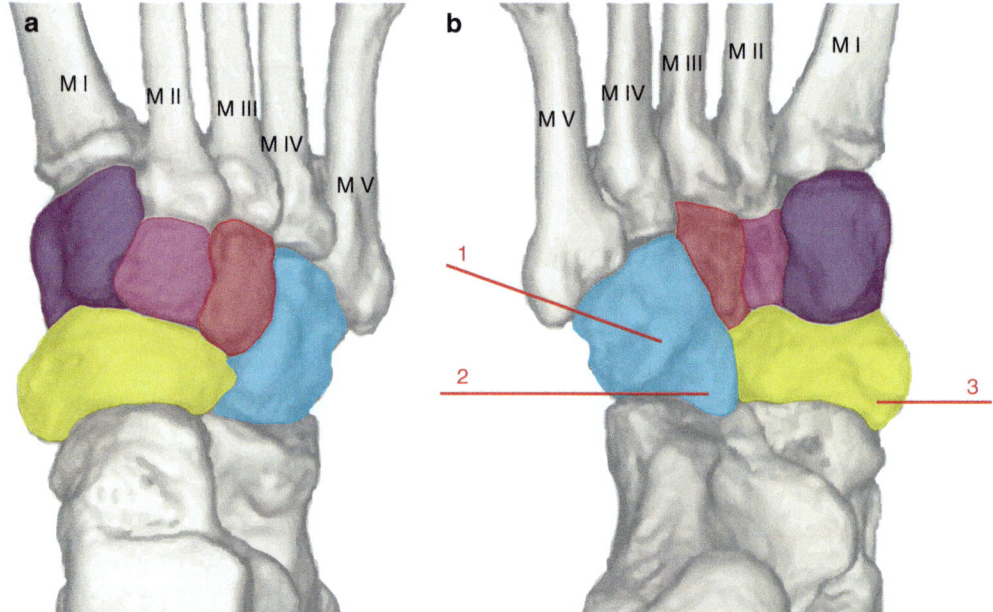

Fig. 23 (**a**, **b**) Anterior tarsus, dorsal view (**a**) and plantar view (**b**). In yellow: navicular. In blue: cuboid. In purple: medial cuneiform. In pink: intermediate cuneiform. In red: lateral cuneiform. (1) Tuberosity of cuboid. (2) Calcaneal process. (3) Tuberosity of navicular

Metatarsals and Phalanges (Figs. 24 and 25)

The **metatarsus** is composed of **five metatarsals**, numbered 1–5 from the medial to the lateral side of the foot.

From back in front, a metatarsal is made up of a base, a body, and a head. The base is articulated with the tarsus behind and the adjacent metatarsal bones on the sides. The head articulates with the proximal phalanx in the front [51, 100].

Characteristics:

– The first metatarsal presents two small cavities on the plantar part of its head, in connection with the two sesamoid bones.

– The fifth metatarsal presents a prolongation at the side part of its base: the **tuberosity of the fifth metatarsal** on which the fibularis brevis (or peroneus brevis) muscle inserts.

The **toes** are composed of **phalanges**.

Toes II to V are composed of three phalanges: proximal (P1), middle (P2), and distal (P3). The **big toe** (or **hallux**) is composed of two phalanges: proximal (P1) and distal (P2, for this toe). From back in front, a phalanx is made up of a base, a body, and a head (like a metatarsal).

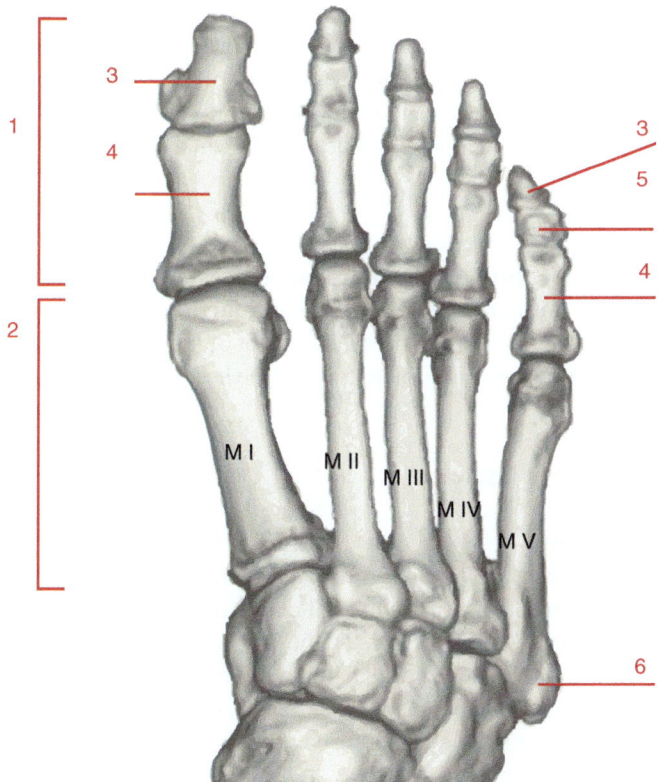

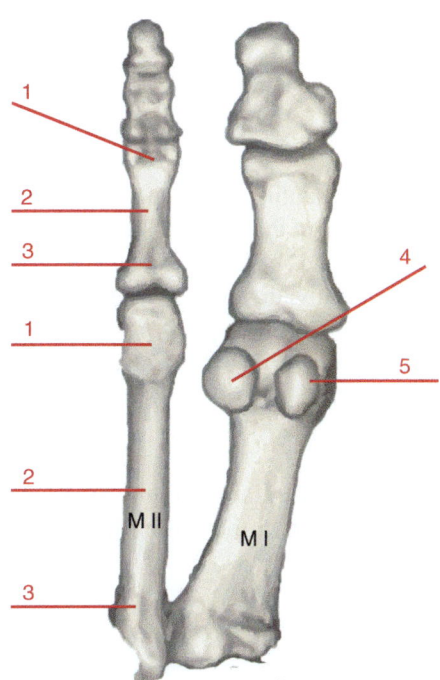

Fig. 25 First and second radius of the foot, plantar view: composition of the metatarsals and the phalanges. (1) Head. (2) Body. (3) Base. (4) Lateral sesamoid. (5) Medial sesamoid

Fig. 24 Metatarsal and phalanges, dorsal view. (1) Toes. (2) Metatarsals. (3) Distal phalanx. (4) Proximal phalanx. (5) Intermediate phalanx. (6) Tuberosity of M5

Sesamoid Bones and Accessory Ossicles
(Fig. 26)

This information comes primarily from Cohen et al. [104] to which the reader can refer for more details.

Definition

- **Sesamoid bone**: Osseous structures developing in a tendon, serving to decrease friction and modify pressure. Some are constant, others not.
- **Accessory ossicles**: Osseous structures not embedded in a tendon. They are inconstant.
- **Supernumerary bones**: Type of accessory ossicles, corresponding to a subdivision of a normal bone or to an osseous prominence separated from the main bone (Table 1) [21, 42, 104, 105].

Sesamoids

Constant:
- **Sesamoids of the hallux**: They are located in the two portions of the tendon of the flexor halluces brevis. There is a lateral sesamoid and a medial sesamoid under the head of the first metatarsal with which they are articulated. They are ossified at around the age of 6 or 7 years. They are frequently bipartite (≈20% of the cases)—primarily the medial sesamoid.

Frequent:
- **Sesamoid of the fibularis longus tendon (os peroneum)**: It is located at the posterolateral and inferior

part of the cuboid (where the tendon of the fibularis longus circumvents the cuboid to pass into a groove on the plantar side of the cuboid). It is articulated with the cuboid. It occurs very frequently (≈25% of patients) but is seldom ossified (1 time out of 5) and is thus visible on X-rays only in approximately 5% of patients. It is bilateral in 60% of cases and can be bipartite.

Not very frequent:
- **Sesamoid of the hallux interphalangeal joint**: It is located under the head of the first phalanx and is articulated with the interphalangeal joint. It is present at 5% of patients.
- **Sesamoid of the tibialis posterior tendon**: It is located close to the tuberosity of navicular (main end point of the tibialis posterior muscle), under the calcaneonavicular ligament (previously: spring ligament). It is present at 5–20% of patients. It should be differentiated from the accessory navicular, which is more distal.
- **Sesamoid of the anterior tibialis anterior tendon**: It is located at the dorsal and medial part of the medial cuneiform (near an insertion point for the tibialis anterior tendon on the medial cuneiform) with which it is generally articulated.

Rare:
- **Sesamoids of the metatarsophalangeal or interphalangeal joints of the second, third, fourth, and fifth toes**: They are located on the plantar facet of the toes, under the foot support zones (mainly under the head of M2 and M5).

Accessory Ossicles

Frequent:
- **Accessory navicular**: A triangular and centimetric bone, developed from an additional center of ossification in the tuberosity of navicular, at the medial extremity of the navicular. It can be articulated with the navicular bone by fibrocartilage (can mimic a fracture), or not be articulated or, more rarely, even be fused with the bone. It is present at 10% of patients.

Not very frequent:
- **Os trigonum**: Located against the lateral tubercle of the posterior process of the talus, with which it is articulated (synchondrosis). It can be fused with the lateral tubercle and gives the elongated lateral process of the talus. It ossifies at around the age of 10 years. It is present at 2–8% of patients. It is often bilateral.
- **Os calcaneus secundarius**: Located above the anterior process of the calcaneus, near the interval between the

Table 1 Frequency of sesamoid bones and accessory ossicles

Sesamoid bones	Accessory bones
Constant: – Of the hallux MTP joint	**Frequent:** – Accessory navicular
Frequent: – Of the fibularis longus tendon (os peroneum)	**Not very fréquent:** – Os trigonum – Os calcaneus secundarius
Not very frequent: – Of the hallux IP joint – Of the tibialis posterior tendon – Of the tibialis anterior tendon	**Rare:** – Os subtibiale – Os subfibulare – Accessory calcaneal
Rare: – Of the MTP or IP joints of the second, third, fourth, and fifth toes	– Os sustentaculi – Os supranaviculare – Os supratalare – Os subcalcis – Os aponeurosis plantaris – Os intermetatarseum – Os vesalianum

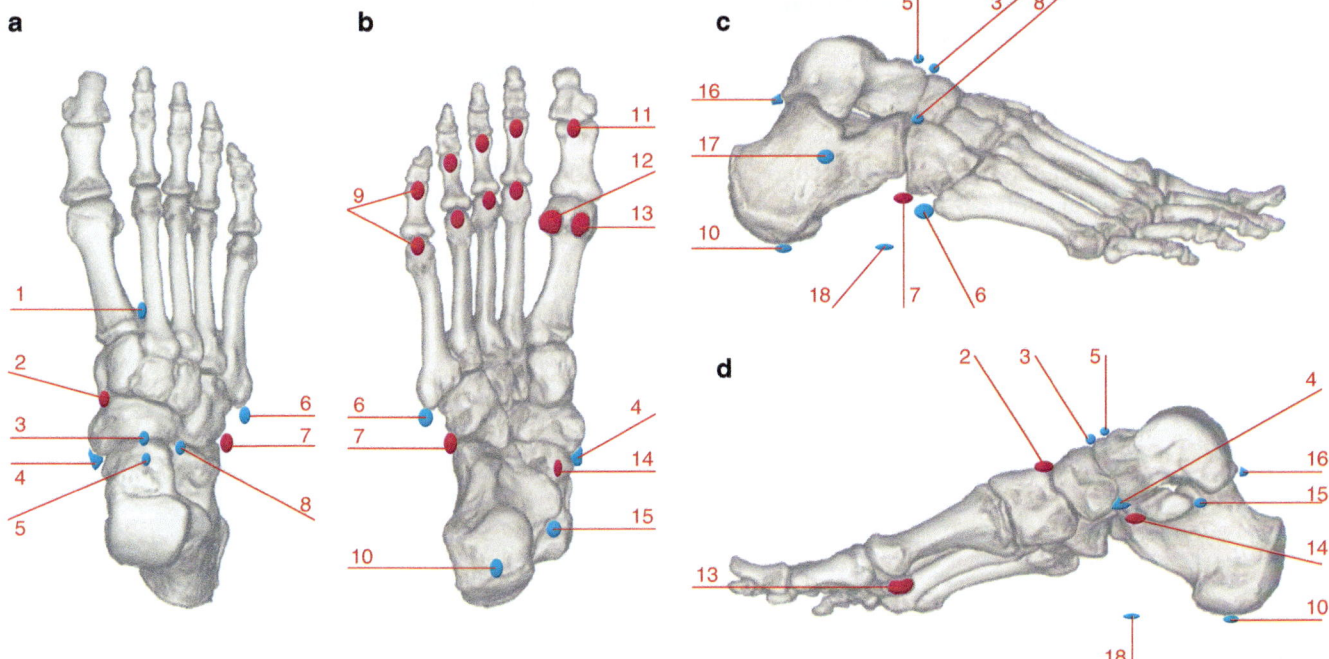

Fig. 26 (**a–d**) Sesamoid bones and accessory ossicles of the foot. Right foot, dorsal (**a**), plantar (**b**), lateral (**c**), and medial views (**d**). In pink: sesamoid bones. In blue: accessory ossicles. (1) Os intermetatarseum. (2) Sesamoid of the tibialis anterior tendon. (3) Os supranaviculare. (4) Accessory navicular. (5) Os supratalare. (6) Os vesalianum. (7) Os peroneum. (8) Calcaneus secundarius. (9) Sesamoids of the MTP or IP of the second, third, fourth, and fifth toes. (10) Os subcalcis. (11) Sesamoid of the hallux PIP. (12) Lateral sesamoid of the hallux. (13) Medial sesamoid of the hallux. (14) Sesamoid of the tibialis posterior tendon. (15) Os sustentaculi. (16) Os trigonum. (17) Accessory calcaneus. (18) Os aponeurosis plantaris

calcaneus, the talus, the navicular bone, and the cuboid bone. It is present at 7 at 10% of teenagers and less than 3% of adults.

Rare:
- **Os subtibiale**: Located under the medial malleolus, on its posterior side
- **Os subfibulare**: Located under the lateral malleolus, on its posterior side
- **Accessory calcaneal**: Located at the lateral surface of the calcaneus, in the prolongation of the lateral malleolus
- **Os sustentaculi**: Located behind the sustentaculum tali and can be articulated with it

- **Os supranaviculare**: Located on the dorsal side of the talonavicular joint space or in contact with the dorsal and proximal edges of the navicular bone
- **Os supratalare**: Located above the head of the talus
- **Os subcalcis**: Located under the plantar side of the calcaneal tuberosity, behind of the insertion of the plantar aponeurosis
- **Os aponeurosis plantaris**: Located in the plantar aponeurosis
- **Os intermetatarseum**: Located between the base of the first and second metatarsal, usually on the dorsal side
- **Os vesalianum**: Located near the base of the fifth metatarsal

Inferior Tibiofibular Joint (or Tibiofibular Syndesmosis) (Figs. 27 and 28)

The tibia and the fibula are firmly jointed from top to bottom by the superior tibiofibular joint, the interosseous membrane of leg (stretching between the tibial and fibular diaphyses), and the inferior tibiofibular joint [51, 103].

The inferior tibiofibular joint is a syndesmosis, without articular cartilage: it joins the lateral edge of the distal tibial epiphysis and the medial edge of the distal fibular epiphysis, above the ankle.

The two bone surfaces are connected by the interosseous ligament. The articulation is maintained in the front by the anterior tibiofibular ligament and behind by the posterior tibiofibular ligament.

The tibiofibular syndesmosis, with its three ligaments, ensures the stability of the tibiofibular mortise.

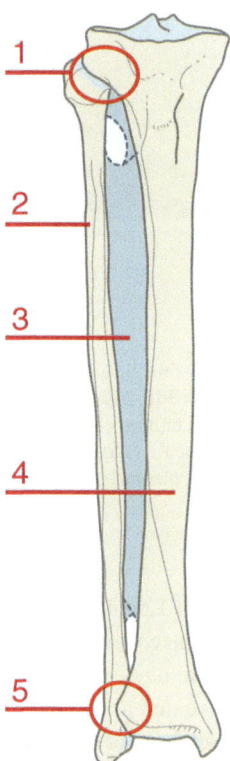

Fig. 27 Tibia and fibula union, anterior view. (1) Superior tibiofibular joint. (2) Fibula. (3) Interosseous membrane of leg. (4) Tibia. (5) Inferior tibiofibular joint

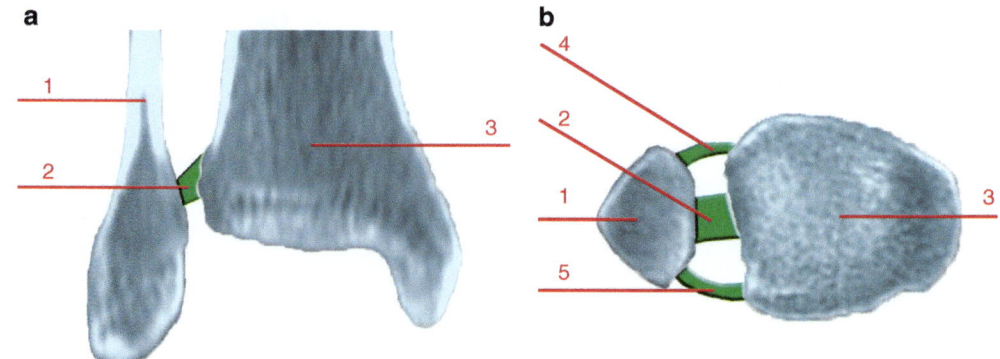

Fig. 28 (**a, b**) Inferior tibiofibular joint, frontal (**a**) and transverse slices (**b**). (1) Fibula. (2) Interosseous ligament. (3) Tibia. (4) Ant. tibiofibular ligament. (5) Post. tibiofibular ligament

Ankle Joint (Fig. 29)

The ankle joint links the tibia, the fibula, and the talus: the trochlea of talus inserts in the tibiofibular mortise. It is a **synovial articulation** allowing the movements of extension (which moves the back of the foot away from the front of the leg) and of flexion [51, 103].

The **tibiofibular mortise** has **three articular surfaces**:

– Inferior articular surface of the tibia
– The articular facet of the medial malleolus (in continuity with the inferior articular surface of the tibia)
– Articular facet of the lateral malleolus

The trochlea of talus has **three continuous articular surfaces**:

– Articular facet of trochlea (talar dome)
– Medial malleolar facet
– Lateral malleolar facet

The thickness of the articular cartilage is greater (approximately 2 mm) on the inferior articular surface of the tibia and the articular facet of the trochlea [51, 103].

The **fibrous membrane of the articular capsule** inserts close to the circumference of cartilaginous surfaces of the ankle joint, except in the front: on the talus, insertion is 1 cm in front, on the neck of the talus; on the tibia, insertion is 7–8 mm above, on the anterior face [51, 103]. This anterior insertion further away from the cartilage allows the joint to open toward the front during extension of ankle (30–60°).

The **synovial membrane of the articular capsule** covers the inner face with the fibrous membrane and the bone through to the circumference of the articular cartilage. The synovial membrane has an upper prolongation between the fibula and the tibia, to the tibiofibular syndesmosis: This prolongation makes it possible to fill the interval which is created between the two bones during certain movements of the ankle joint [103].

The ligaments that support the joint will be treated later in the book.

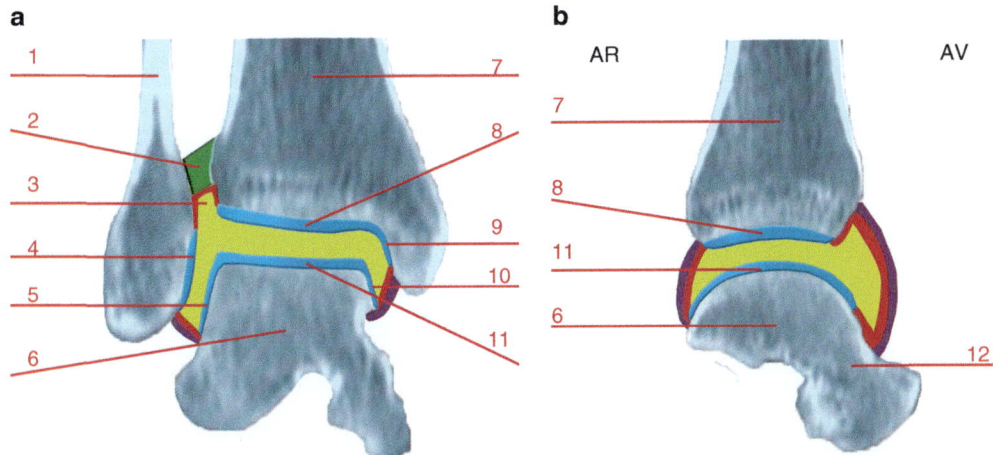

Fig. 29 (**a**, **b**) Ankle joint, frontal (**a**) and sagittal slices (**b**). In red: synovial membrane of the articular capsule. In purple: fibrous membrane of the articular capsule. In blue: articular cartilage. In yellow: synovial fluid. In green: ligament. (1) Fibula. (2) Interosseous ligament. (3) Cul-de-sac of the synovial membrane. (4) Articular facet of the lateral malleolus. (5) Lateral malleolar facet. (6) Talus. (7) Tibia. (8) Inferior articular surface of the tibia. (9) Articular facet of the medial malleolus. (10) Medial malleolar facet. (11) Articular facet of trochlea of the talus. (12) Neck of the talus

Subtalar Joint (Talocalcaneal Joint) (Fig. 30)

The subtalar joint links the talus and the calcaneus, behind the sinus tarsi.

The posterior talar articular surface articulates with the posterior calcaneal articular surface.

This synovial joint has its own articular capsule and is maintained by the medial, lateral, posterior, and interosseous talocalcaneal ligaments: Talocalcaneal interosseous ligament is short and very resistant and composed of two fibrous bands stretched vertically in the sinus tarsi [51, 100, 103].

The subtalar joint enables eversion-inversion foot movements (adapting the foot position on rough ground).

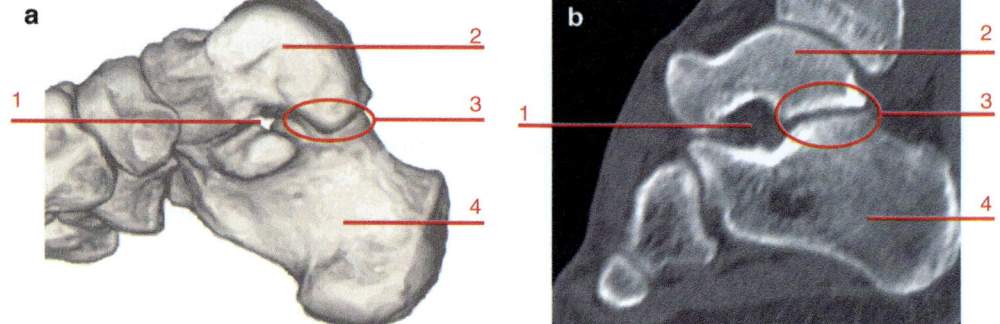

Fig. 30 (**a, b**) Subtalar joint, medial view (**a**) and sagittal CT slice (**b**). (1) Sinus tarsi. (2) Talus. (3) Subtalar joint. (4) Calcaneus

Transverse Tarsal Joint
(Chopart Joint) (Figs. 31, 32, and 33)

The transverse tarsal joint links the anterior tarsus and the posterior tarsus.

The transverse tarsal joint is made up of two articulations:

– The talocalcaneonavicular joint medially
– The calcaneocuboid joint laterally

The **talocalcaneonavicular joint** links the head of the talus, the navicular in the front, and the anterosuperior part of the calcaneus below.

It is a synovial articulation with its own articular capsule: the articulation between the anterior part of the head of the talus and the navicular is in continuity with the anterior and middle talocalcaneal joints (in front of the sinus tarsi).

Medially, the **plantar calcaneonavicular ligament** (calcaneonavicular ligament, spring ligament) helps support the head of the talus. The plantar calcaneonavicular ligament stretches like a hammock from the sustentaculum tali to the plantar edge of the navicular: its dorsal part is encrusted with cartilage, articulates with the head of the talus, and takes part in the talocalcaneonavicular joint [51].

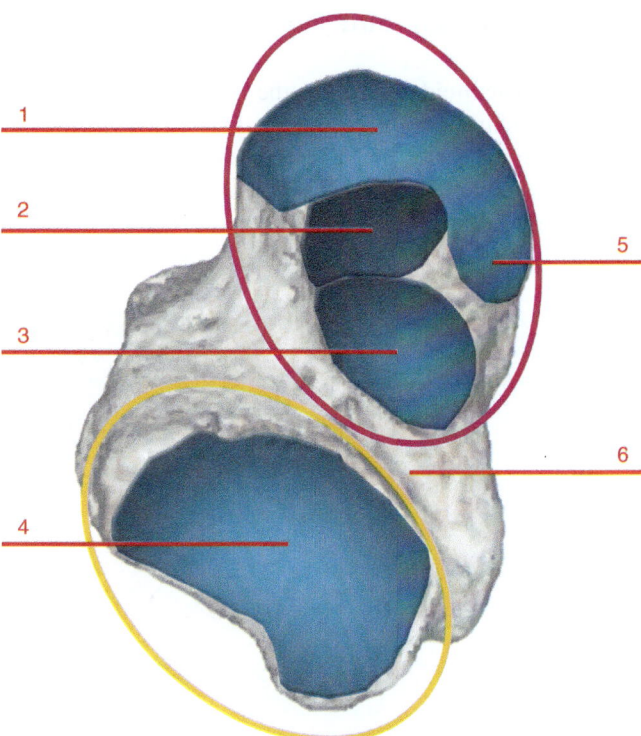

Fig. 32 Talocalcaneonavicular joint: talus, plantar view. Pink outline: participated in the talocalcaneonavicular joint. Yellow outline: participates in the subtalar joint. (1) Navicular articular surface. (2) Ant. calcaneal articular surface. (3) Middle calcaneal articular surface. (4) Post. calcaneal articular surface. (5) Articular surface of the plantar calcaneonavicular ligament. (6) Talar sulcus

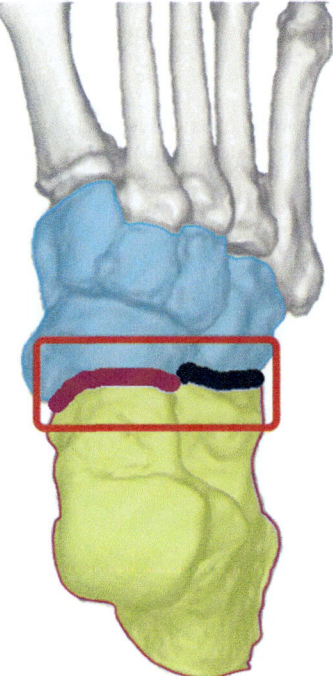

Fig. 31 Transverse tarsal joint, dorsal view. In yellow: posterior tarsus. In blue: anterior tarsus. Pink line: talocalcaneonavicular joint. Black line: calcaneocuboid joint. Red box: transverse tarsal joint

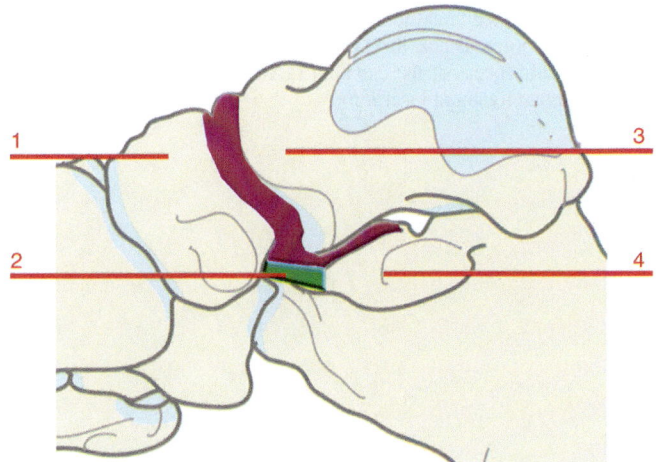

Fig. 33 Talocalcaneonavicular joint: medial view. In pink: talocalcaneonavicular joint. (1) Navicular. (2) Plantar calcaneonavicular ligament. (3) Head of the talus. (4) Sustentaculum tali

Transverse Tarsal Joint (Figs. 34 and 35)

The **calcaneocuboid joint** links the anterior process of the calcaneus behind and the cuboid in front. It is a synovial articulation with its own articular capsule. On top the anterior process of the calcaneus overhangs it, and underneath, it is supported by the calcaneal process of the cuboid.

The talocalcaneonavicular and calcaneocuboid joints are distinctive but have the calcaneus in common and are connected by the solid **bifurcate ligament**. The bifurcate ligament is dorsal, fits behind on the deep hollow on the upper surface of the calcaneus, and sends out two anterior bands, one for the cuboid and the other for the navicular.

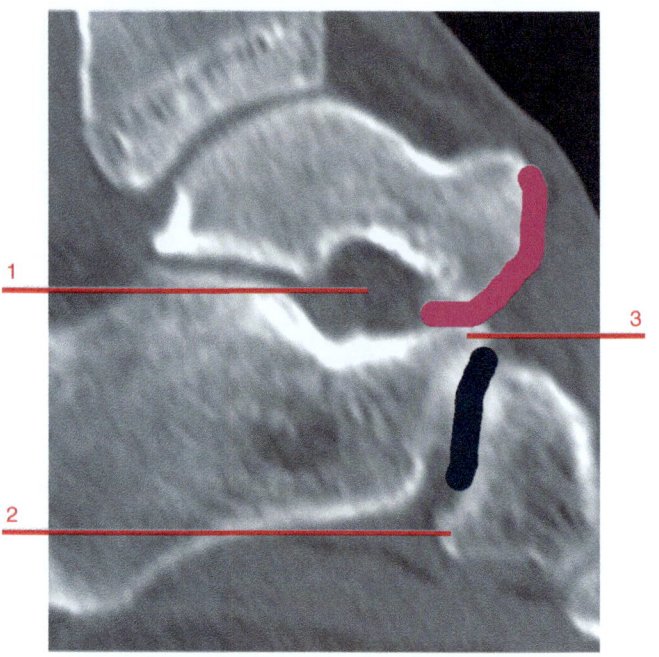

Fig. 34 Transverse tarsal joint, sagittal CT slice. Pink line: talocalcaneonavicular joint. Black line: calcaneocuboid joint. (1) Sinus tarsi. (2) Calcaneal process of the cuboid. (3) Anterior process of the calcaneus (bifurcate ligament insertion)

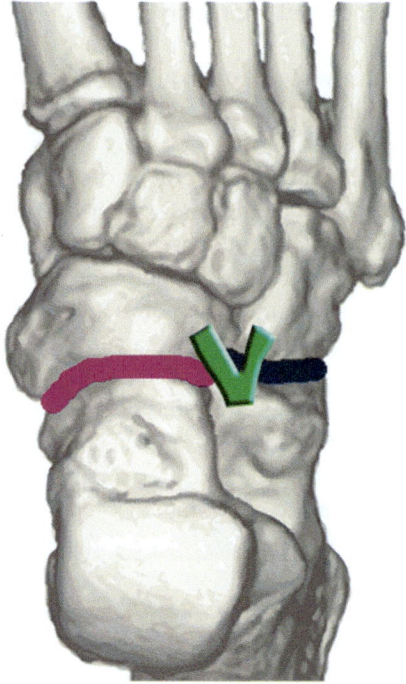

Fig. 35 Bifurcate ligament, dorsal view. Pink line: talocalcaneonavicular joint. Black line: calcaneocuboid joint. In green: bifurcate ligament

Anterior Tarsal Bone Joints and Tarsometatarsal Joints (Figs. 36 and 37)

Anterior tarsal bone joints

They link the navicular, the cuboid, and the three cuneiforms.

There are five synovial articulations [51, 103]:

– The cuneonavicular joint between the navicular in the back and the three cuneiforms in the front
– The two medial and lateral intercuneiform joints
– The cuboid-navicular joint (often a syndesmosis [51])
– The cuneocuboid joint

The synovial cavity of the cuneonavicular joint often communicates with the other joints of the anterior tarsus.

Tarsometatarsal joints (Lisfranc joint)

They link the three cuneiforms and the cuboid behind and the base of the five metatarsal bones in the front.

There are three synovial articulations [51, 103]:

– The medial tarsometatarsal joint, between the medial cuneiform and M1
– The intermediate tarsometatarsal joint, between the intermediary and lateral cuneiforms and M2 and M3
– The lateral tarsometatarsal joint, between the cuboid and M4 and M5

The medial tarsometatarsal joint has an independent synovial cavity. It is important to examine the medial tarsometatarsal joint prior to surgery of the first metatarsophalangeal joint for hallux valgus.

The tarsometatarsal joints form an oblique space on the outside back. This space is irregular, with in particular the base of the second metatarsal which inserts behind in the mortise created by the three cuneiforms [103].

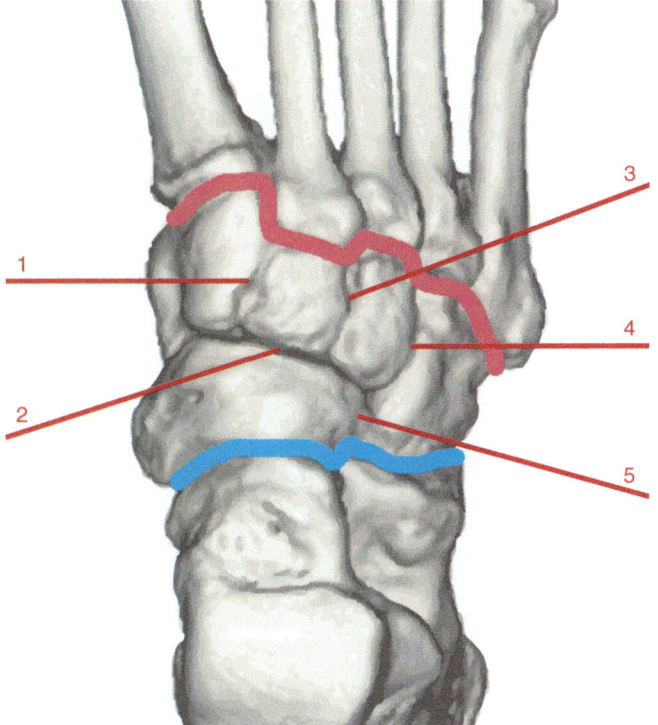

Fig. 36 Articulations of the anterior tarsal bones, dorsal view. Pink line: tarsometatarsal joints. Blue line: transverse tarsal joint. (1) Medial intercuneiform joint. (2) Cuneonavicular joint. (3) Lateral intercuneiform joint. (4) Cuneocuboid joint. (5) Cuboid-navicular joint

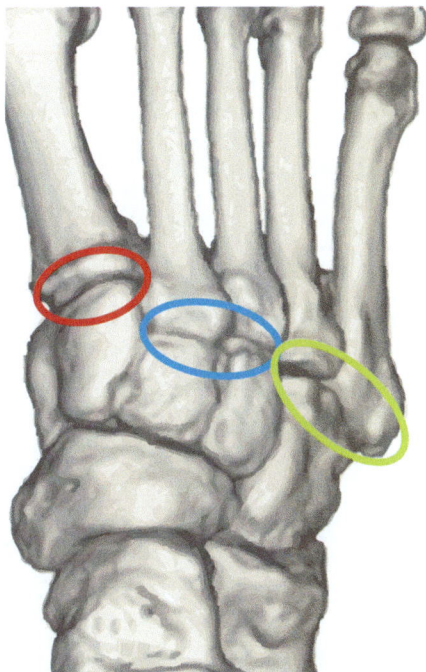

Fig. 37 Tarsometatarsal joints, dorsal view. Red box: medial tarsometatarsal joint. Blue box: intermediary tarsometatarsal joint. Yellow box: lateral tarsometatarsal joint

Intermetatarsal, Metatarsophalangeal, and Interphalangeal Joints (Figs. 38 and 39)

Intermetatarsal joints

The metatarsals are articulated between themselves by their base.

The intermetatarsal joints are synovial (except the articulation between M1 and M2 which is a syndesmosis), often in continuity with the tarsometatarsal joints.

Metatarsophalangeal joints

They link the head of a metatarsal and the base of a proximal phalanx.

They are synovial articulations.

The articular capsule is thin at the back, which fits into the circumference of the articular cartilage. The plantar part is thicker, fits into the circumference of the cartilage of the base of the phalanx, but is further behind the cartilage of the head of the metatarsal: The inner side is lined with fibrocartilage of the labrum type which prolongs below and behind the articulation.

The plantar surface of the head of M1 articulates with the two medial and lateral sesamoids, included in the fibrocartilage of the articular capsule [21, 51].

Interphalangeal joints

They link the base and the head of two successive phalanx [51].

There are two interphalangeal joints—proximal and distal—for each toe, except for the hallux which has only one interphalangeal joint [103].

They are synovial articulations.

The articular capsule is identical to that of the metatarsophalangeal articulations.

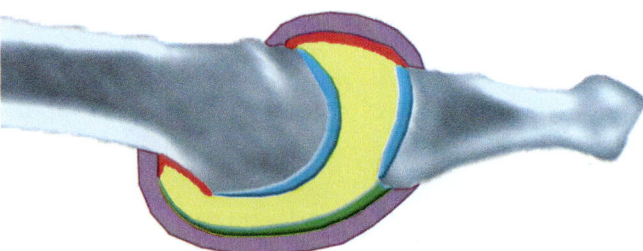

Fig. 39 Metatarsophalangeal joint, sagittal slice. In red: synovial membrane of the articular capsule. In purple: fibrous membrane of the articular capsule. In blue: articular cartilage. In yellow: synovial fluid. In green: fibrocartilage

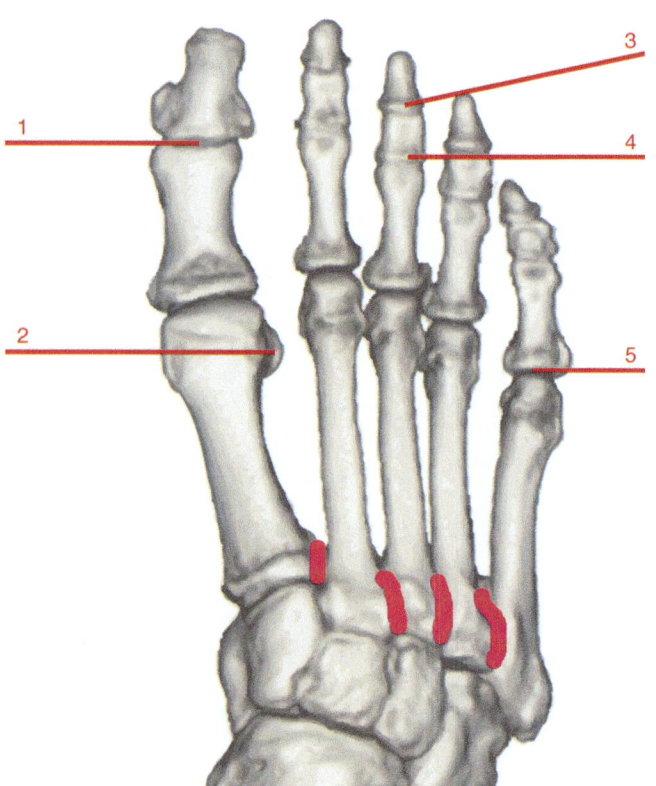

Fig. 38 Toe joints, dorsal view. Pink lines: intermetatarsal joints. (1) Hallux interphalangeal joint. (2) Lateral sesamoid. (3) Distal interphalangeal joint of the third ray. (4) Proximal interphalangeal joint of the third ray. (5) Metatarsophalangeal joint of the fifth ray

Ligaments of the Ankle (Figs. 40 and 41)

The talocrural joint is supported by two powerful ligaments [51]:

- The medial collateral ligament (or deltoid ligament)
- The lateral collateral ligament

The **medial collateral ligament** is triangular, is composed of four bands in two layers, and fits in proximally on the apex of the medial malleolus:

- Surface layer: extends in two bands toward the navicular and the calcaneus

- Inner layer: extends onto the talus in two anterior and posterior tibiotalar bands

The **lateral collateral ligament** is composed of three bands in only one layer and fits in proximally on the lateral malleolus and distally on:

- The talus: two talofibular bands, anterior and posterior
- The calcaneus: one calcaneofibular band

The anterior talofibular ligament is the first ligament impacted with a traditional ankle varus sprain.

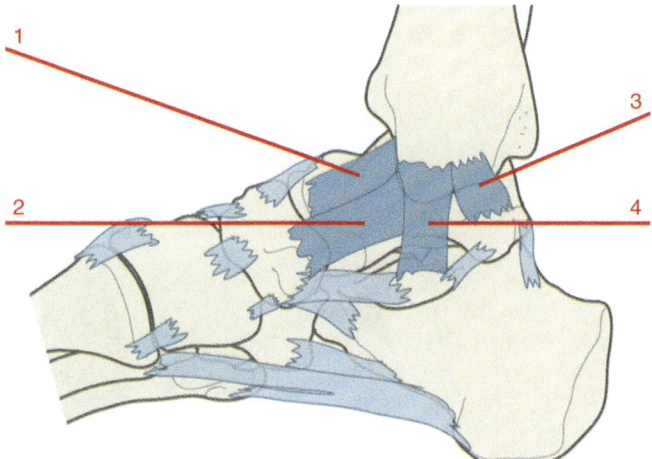

Fig. 40 Medial collateral ligament. (1) Ant. tibiotalar ligament. (2) Tibionavicular ligament. (3) Post. tibiotalar ligament. (4) Tibiocalcaneal ligament

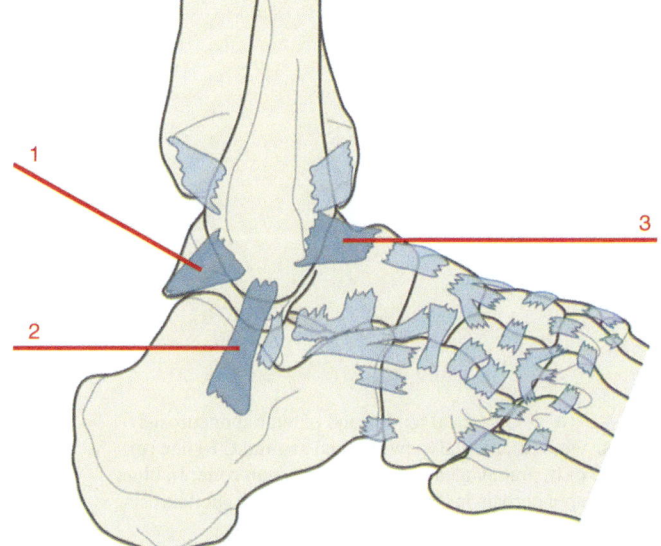

Fig. 41 Lateral collateral ligament. (1) Post. talofibular ligament. (2) Calcaneofibular ligament. (3) Ant. talofibular ligament

Calcaneal Tendon and Plantar Aponeurosis (Fig. 42)

Calcaneal tendon [51, 100, 103]:
It is the largest tendon of the body. It connects the triceps surae muscle to the mid-third posterior part of the calcaneal tuberosity. The synovial bursa of the calcaneal tendon, located between the calcaneal tendon and the calcaneus, protects the tendon from the movements of friction.

Plantar aponeurosis [51, 100, 103]:
This is a very resistant surface band, corresponding to a thickening of the plantar fascia. The plantar aponeurosis is triangular: its top is posterior and inserts on the plantar part of the calcaneal tuberosity. Its anterior base finishes at the level of the metatarsophalangeal joints in five fibrous strips. The plantar aponeurosis plays a role in maintaining the longitudinal arch of foot.

Extensor system of the foot:
The surface fibers of the calcaneal tendon continue, slipping under the calcaneal tuberosity and mixing with the surface fibers with the plantar aponeurosis [21]. The plantar aponeurosis contributes to propulsion, thanks to the extensor system of the foot.

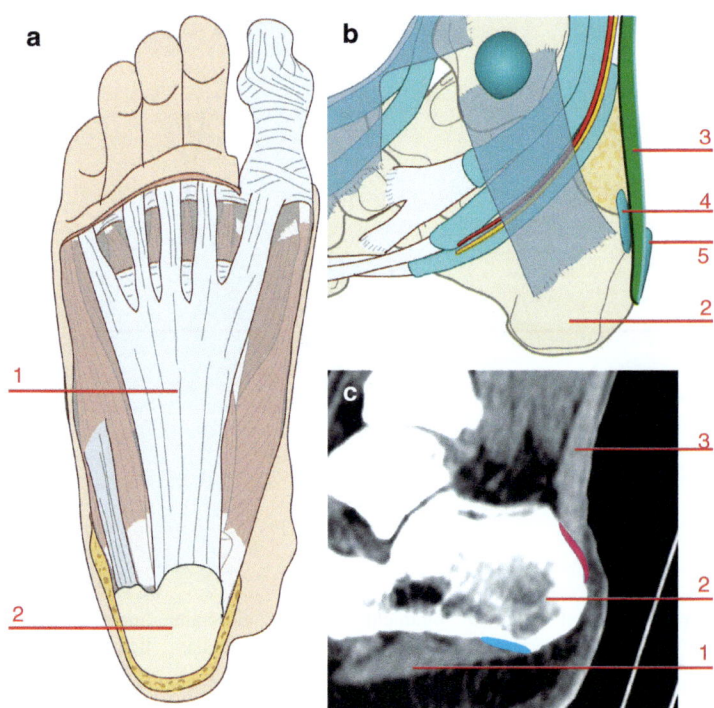

Fig. 42 (**a–c**) Calcaneal tendon and plantar aponeurosis: plantar view (**a**), medial view (**b**), and sagittal CT slice (**c**). (Image **c**) In pink: Calcaneal tendon insertion zone; In blue: Plantar aponeurosis insertion zone. (1) Plantar aponeurosis. (2) Calcaneal tuberosity. (3) Calcaneal tendon. (4) Bursa of calcaneal tendon. (5) Subcutaneous calcaneal bursa

Tendinous Sheaths of the Ankle (Fig. 43)

The muscles of the ankle and of the foot are powerful, and their tendons pass via the ankle, requiring that they be protected by tendinous sheaths (cf. page tendons and aponeuroses).

The tendinous sheaths of the ankle are divided into anterior, lateral, and medial sheaths [51, 100].

The anterior tendinous sheaths of the ankle spread to the front of the ankle and on the dorsal face of the tarsus to the tarsometatarsal joints. They are covered with the superior and inferior extensor retinaculum. They include, inside and outside:

– The TS of tibialis anterior
– The TS of extensor hallucis longus
– The TS of extensor digitorum longus

The medial tendinous sheaths of the ankle extend back ant to the lower part from the medial malleolus and on the medial edge of the tarsus. They are covered with the flexor retinaculum. They include:

– The TS of tibialis posterior
– The TS of flexor hallucis longus
– The TS of flexor digitorum longus

The lateral tendinous sheath of the ankle extends behind and to the lower part from the lateral malleolus to the cuboid bone. It is covered with the superior and inferior fibular retinaculum. It includes:

– The common TS of fibularis brevis and longus

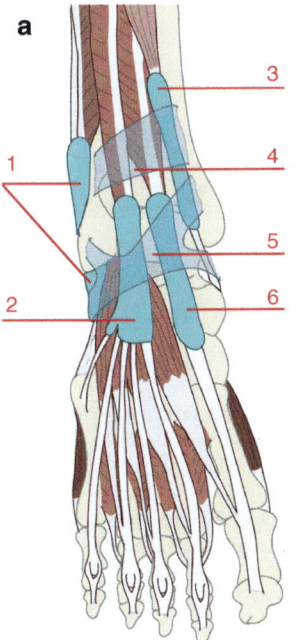
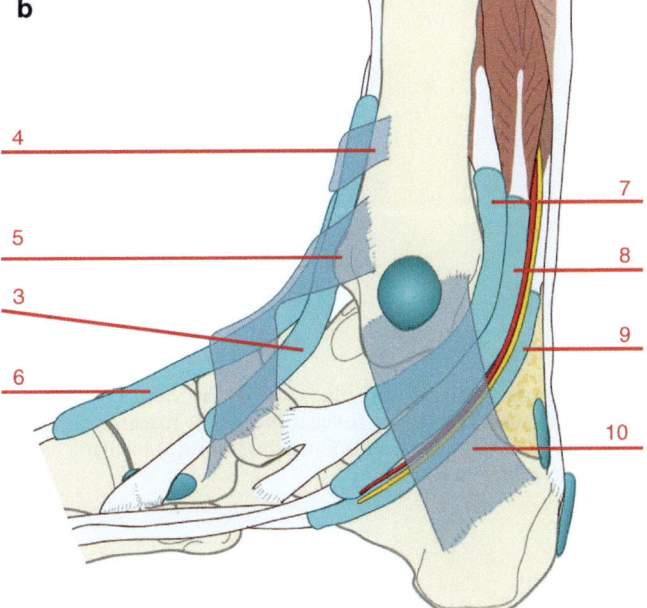

Fig. 43 (**a, b**) Tendinous sheaths (TS) and ankle retinaculum, anterior (**a**) and medial view (**b**). (1) Common TS of fibulares. (2) TS of extensor digitorum longus. (3) TS of tibialis ant. (4) Sup. extensor retinaculum. (5) Inf. extensor retinaculum. (6) TS of extensor hallucis longus. (7) TS of tibialis post. (8) TS of flexor digitorum longus. (9) TS of flexor hallucis longus. (10) Flexor retinaculum

Muscle and Ligament Insertions of the Foot,
Dorsal View (Figs. 44 and 45)

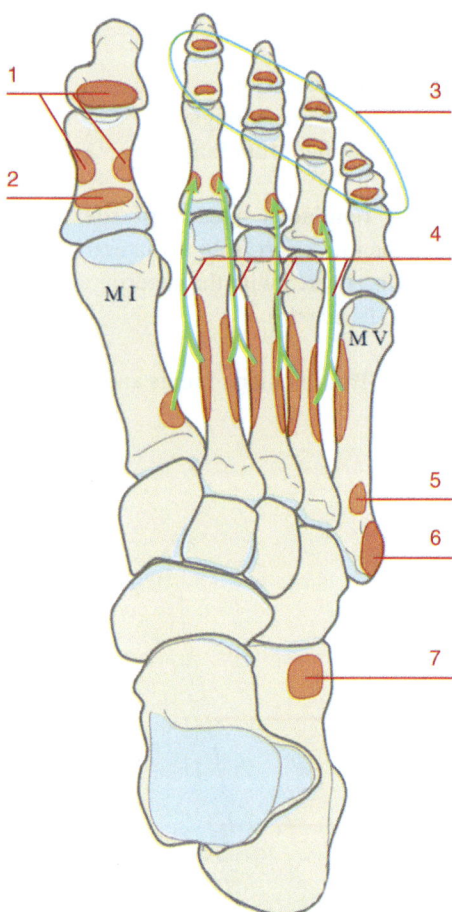

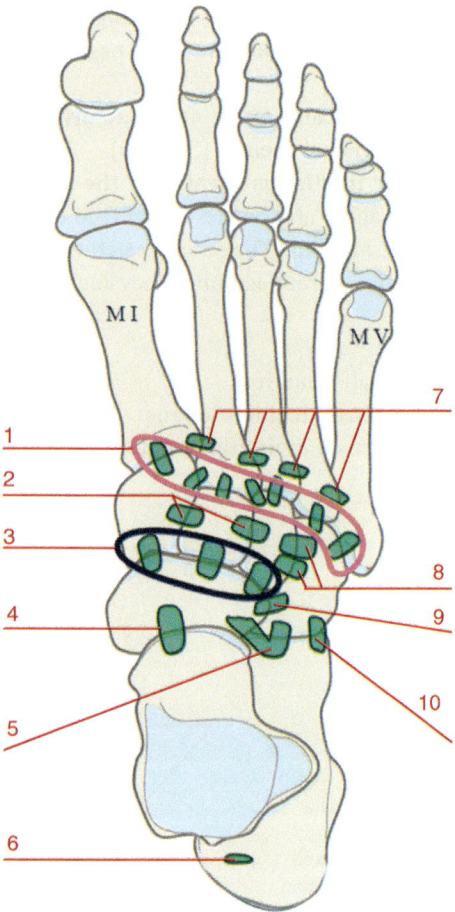

Fig. 44 Muscle insertions of the foot, dorsal view. (1) Extensor halluc1s longus. (2) Extensor halluces brevis. (3) Extensor digitorum longus. (4) Dorsal interossei. (5) Fibularis tertius. (6) Fibularis brevis. (7) Extensor digitorum brevis

Fig. 45 Ligament insertions of the foot, dorsal view. (1) Dorsal tarso-metatarsal ligament. (2) Dorsal intercuneiform ligament. (3) Dorsal cuneonavicular ligament. (4) Talonavicular ligament. (5) Bifurcate ligament. (6) Post. talocalcaneal ligament. (7) Dorsal metatarsal ligament. (8) Dorsal cuneocuboid ligament. (9) Dorsal cuboideonavicular ligament. (10) Dorsal calcaneocuboid ligament

Muscle and Ligament Insertions of the Foot, Plantar View (Figs. 46 and 47)

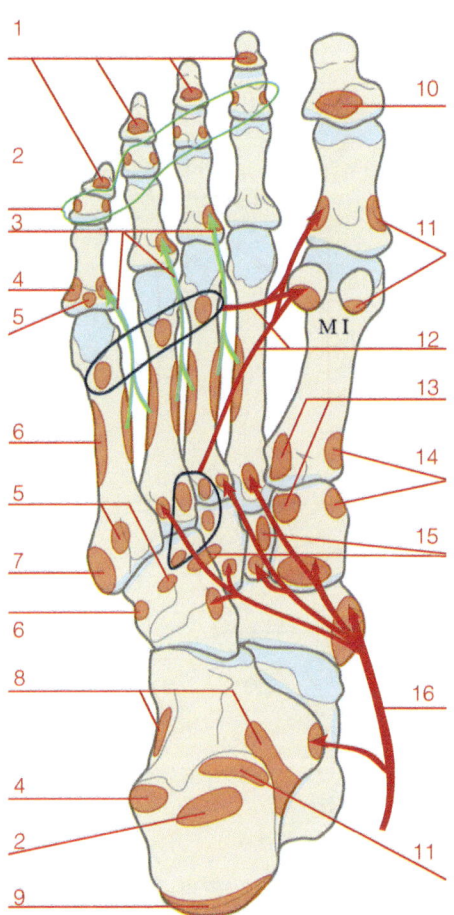

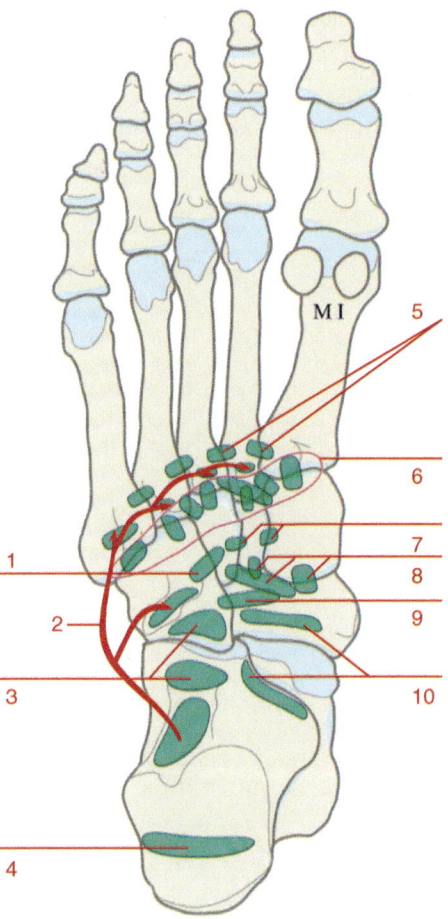

Fig. 46 Muscle insertions of the foot, plantar view. (1) Flexor digitorum longus. (2) Flexor digitorum brevis. (3) Plantar interossei. (4) Abductor digiti minimi. (5) Flexor digiti minimi brevis. (6) Opponens digiti minimi. (7) Fibularis brevis. (8) Quadratus plantae. (9) Calcaneal tendon. (10) Flexor halluces longus. (11) Abductor hallucis. (12) Adductor hallucis. (13) Fibularis longus. (14) Tibialis ant. (15) Flexor hallucis brevis. (16) Tibialis post

Fig. 47 Ligament insertions of the foot, plantar view. (1) Plantar cuneocuboid ligament. (2) Long plantar ligament. (3) Plantar calcaneocuboid ligament. (4) Plantar aponeurosis. (5) Plantar metatarsal ligament. (6) Plantar tarsometatarsal ligament. (7) Plantar intercuneiform ligament. (8) Plantar cuneonavicular ligament. (9) Plantar cuboideonavicular ligament. (10) Plantar calcaneonavicular ligament (spring ligament)

Muscle and Ligament Insertions of the Foot, Medial View (Figs. 48 and 49)

Fig. 48 Muscle insertions of the foot, medial view.
(1) Abductor hallucis.
(2) Tibialis ant. (3) Tibialis post. (4) Quadratus plantae.
(5) Calcaneal tendon

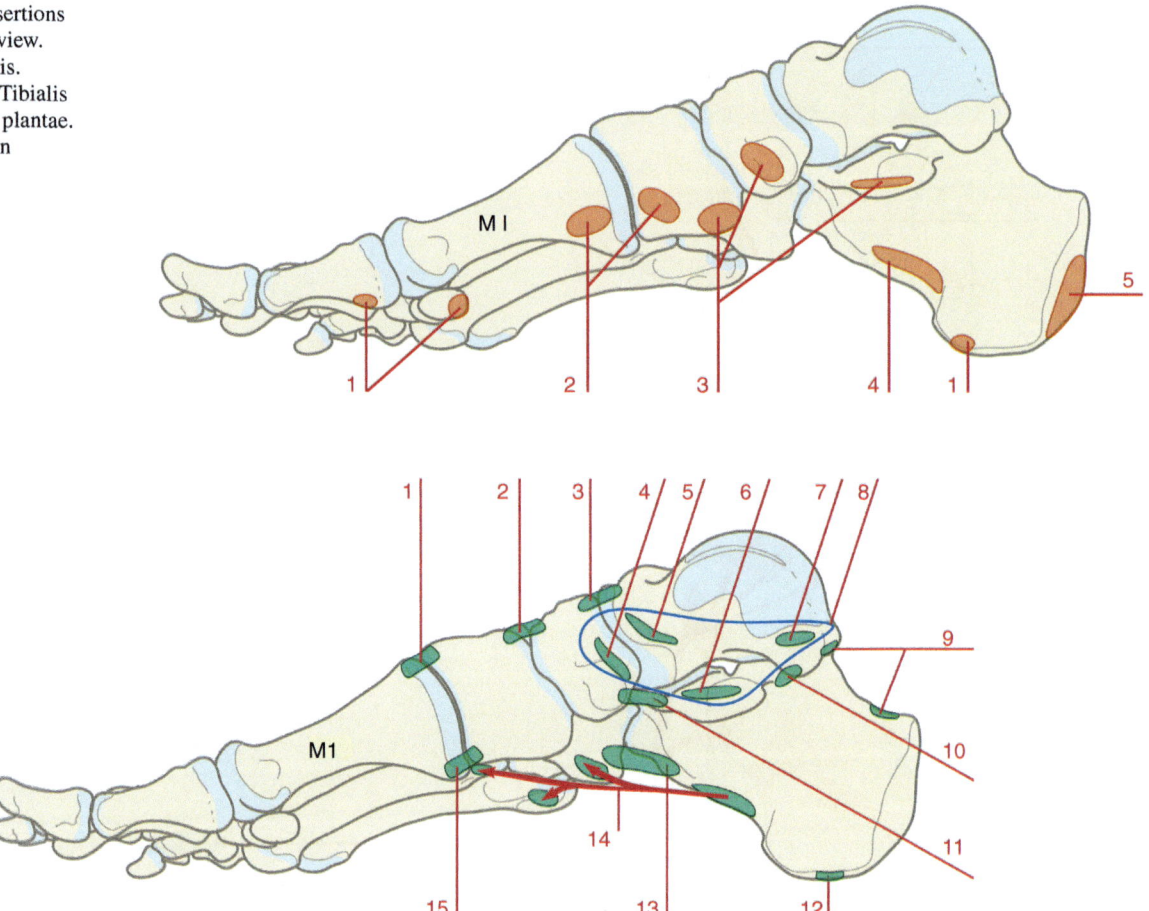

Fig. 49 Ligament insertions of the foot, medial view. (1) Dorsal tarsometatarsal ligament. (2) Dorsal cuneonavicular ligament. (3) Talonavicular ligament. (4) Tibionavicular ligament. (5) Ant. tibiotalar ligament. (6) Tibiocalcaneal ligament. (7) Post. tibiotalar ligament. (8) Medial collateral ligament. (9) Post. talocalcaneal ligament. (10) Medial talocalcaneal ligament. (11) Plantar calcaneonavicular ligament (spring ligament). (12) Plantar aponeurosis. (13) Plantar calcaneocuboid ligament. (14) Long plantar ligament. (15) Plantar tarsometatarsal ligament

Muscle and Ligament Insertions of the Foot, Lateral View (Figs. 50 and 51)

Fig. 50 Muscle insertions of the foot, lateral view.
(1) Extensor digitorum brevis.
(2) Calcaneal tendon.
(3) Abductor digiti minimi.
(4) Quadratus plantae.
(5) Opponens digiti minimi.
(6) Fibularis brevis.
(7) Fibularis tertius

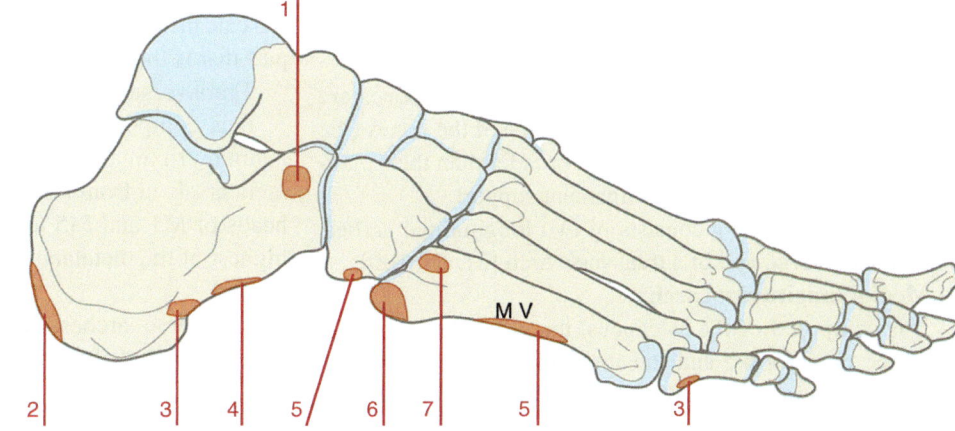

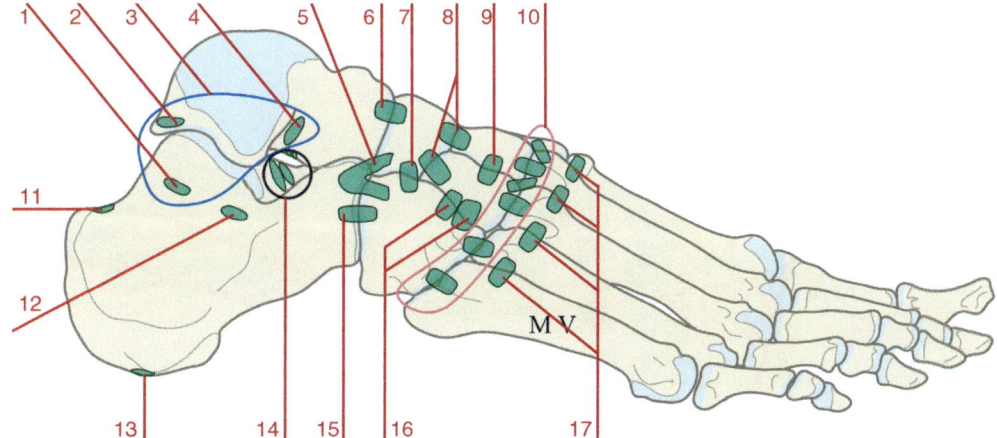

Fig. 51 Ligament insertions of the foot, lateral view. (1) Calcaneofibular ligament. (2) Post. talofibular ligament. (3) Lateral collateral ligament. (4) Ant. talofibular ligament. (5) Bifurcate ligament. (6) Talonavicular ligament. (7) Dorsal cuboideonavicular ligament. (8) Dorsal cuneonavicular ligament. (9) Dorsal intercuneiform ligament. (10) Dorsal tarsometatarsal ligament. (11) Posterior talocalcaneal ligament. (12) Inf. fibular retinaculum. (13) Plantar aponeurosis. (14) Talocalcaneal interosseous ligament. (15) Dorsal calcaneocuboid ligament. (16) Dorsal cuneocuboid ligament. (17) Dorsal metatarsal ligament

Arch of the Foot and Points of Support
(Figs. 52 and 53)

The plantar surface of the foot forms an arch. This arch, combined with the viscoelastic capacities with the foot, ensures support and propulsion with minimum effort.

The arch of the foot stems from how the tarsal bones are positioned among themselves, by the shape of the bones (the cuneiforms have a dorsal side that is broader than their plantar side) and by tendinous and ligament support.

The arch of the foot consists of two longitudinal arches, medial and lateral, and of a transverse arch [21, 51, 100].

Medial longitudinal arch:

It is composed of the calcaneus, the talus, the navicular, the three cuneiforms, and the three first metatarsals. This arch continues in the front of the foot with the first three toes, forming the talar propulsive part of the foot (the most flexible and mobile part). The articulations of this arch are the most used and the most often affected by osteoarthritis.

Lateral longitudinal arch:

Lower than the medial longitudinal arch, it is composed of the calcaneus, the cuboid, and the two last metatarsals. This arch continues forward with the last two toes to form the calcaneal weight-bearing part of the foot (the most static part that is the most often in contact with the ground).

Transversal arch:

It is composed of the five bones of the anterior tarsus behind (proximal transverse arch of foot) and the head of the metatarsals in front (distal transverse arch of foot). Only the heads of M1 and M5 touch the ground. The head of M2 is highest of the metatarsal heads, approximately 9 mm off the ground.

The three arches determine the **three main weight-bearing points** of the foot:

- Tuberosity of calcaneus in the back (main fulcrum)
- Heads of M1 and M5 in the front

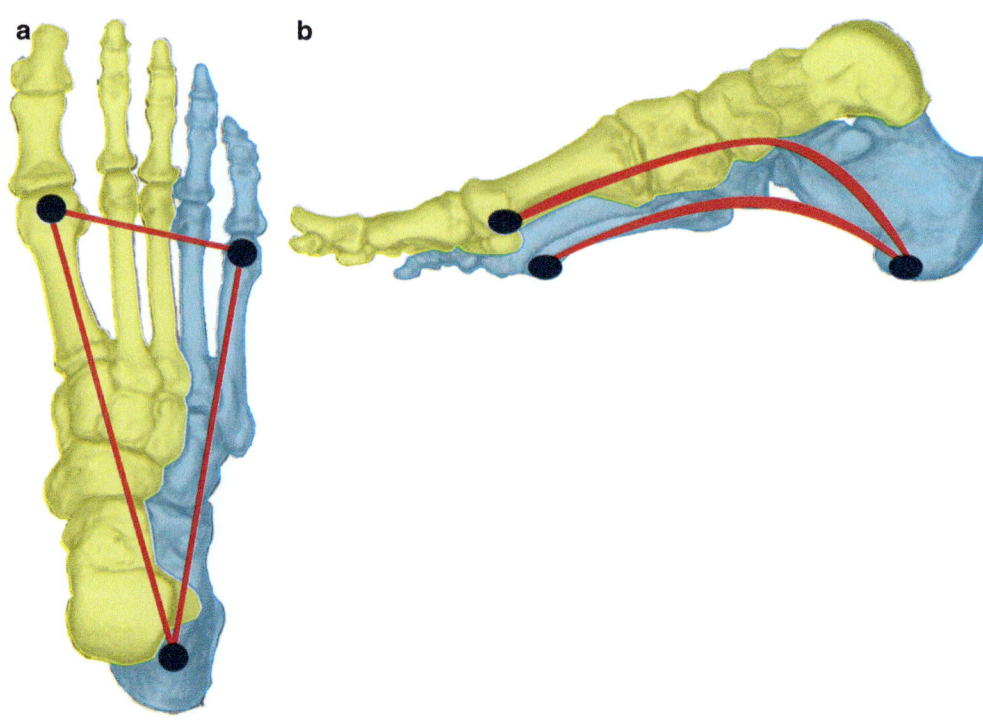

Fig. 52 (**a, b**) Arches and points of support of the foot, dorsal (**a**) and medial view (**b**). In yellow: propelling talar foot. In blue: calcaneal weight-bearing foot. Red lines: arches of the foot. Black spots: plantar points or support

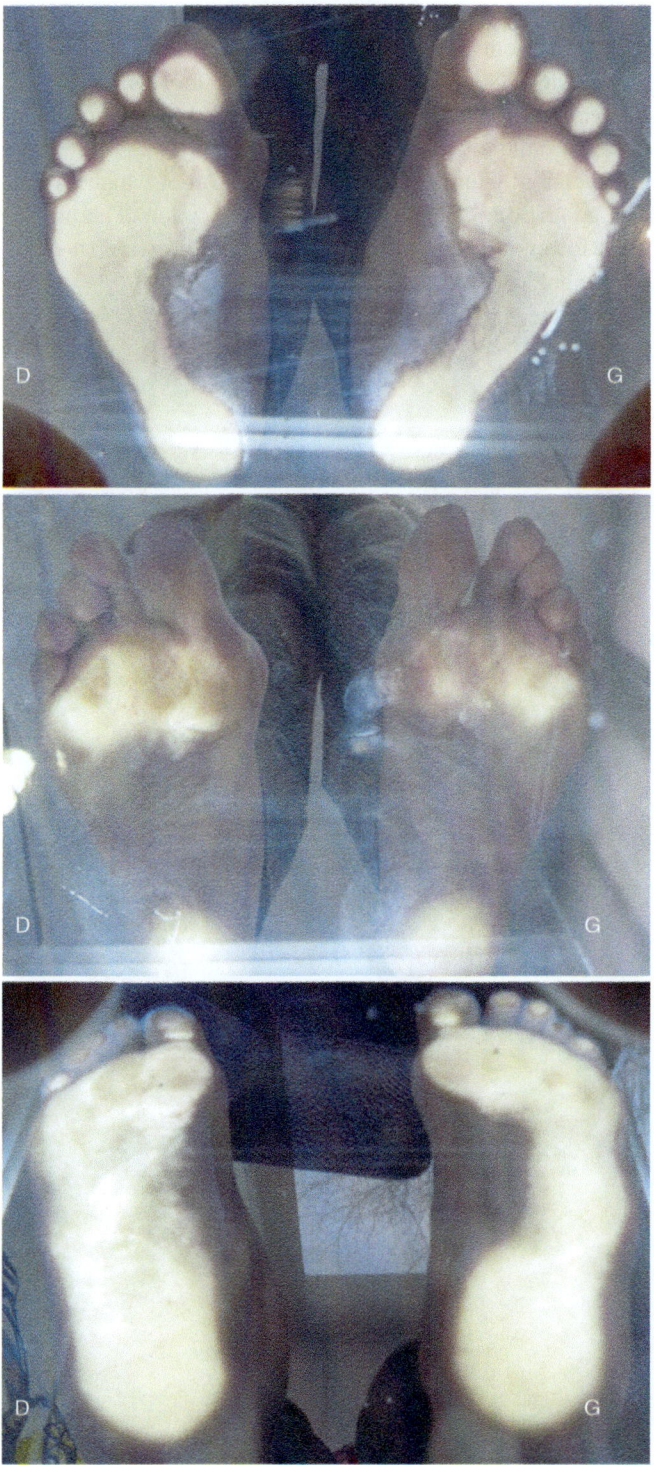

Fig. 53 (**a–c**) Podoscope: normal feet (**a**), bilateral cavus feet (**b**), and right flatfoot (**c**)

Movements of the Foot (Fig. 54)

Flexion: Movement that closes the joint.

Extension: Movement that opens the joint.

Abduction (or valgus): Movement around a sagittal axis that moves a segment of the limb away from the medial plane.

Adduction (or varus): Movement around a sagittal axis that brings a segment of the limb closer to the median plane.

Lateral rotation: Movement around a vertical axis which turns a segment clockwise (for a right limb).

Medial rotation: Movement around a vertical axis that turns a segment counterclockwise (for a right limb).

Eversion: Complex movement of the foot which associates abduction, flexion, and lateral rotation. This movement raises the sole of the foot up and out.

Inversion: Complex movement of the foot which associates adduction, extension, and medial rotation. This movement lowers the sole of the foot down and inward (it is the classic ankle sprain movement).

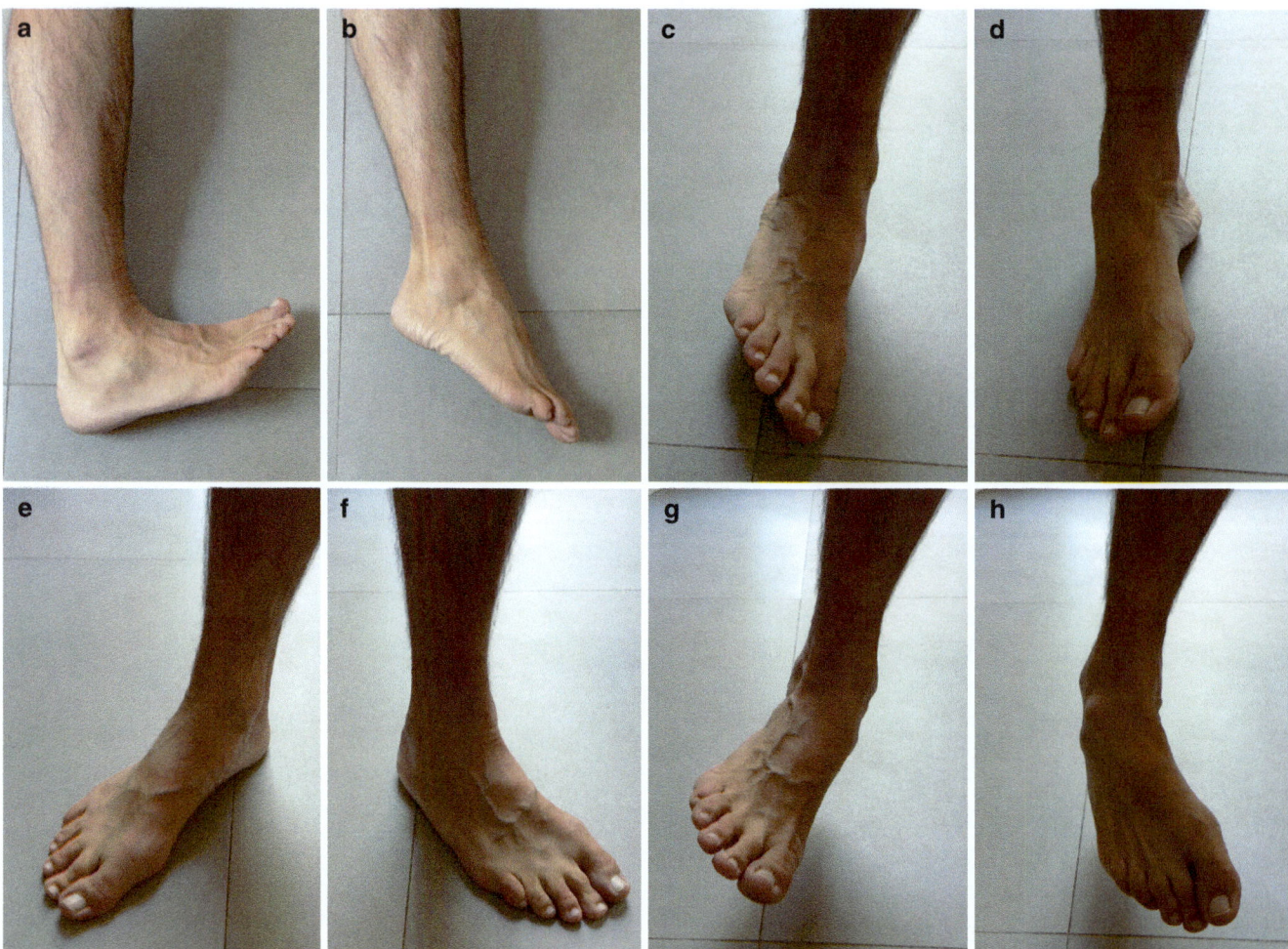

Fig. 54 Movements of the right foot: flexion (**a**), extension (**b**), abduction (**c**), adduction (**d**), lateral rotation (**e**), medial rotation (**f**), eversion (**g**), and inversion (**h**)

Appendix

Biomaterials

Definition:
- "A material intended to interface with biological systems to evaluate, treat, augment, or replace any tissue, organ, or function of the body." (Chester conference, 1991)
- A biomaterial must be biocompatible (nontoxic and not degraded by the body) and biofunctional (totally adapted to each clinical usage).
- In orthopedics, biomaterials are used for the **bone grafts**, **osteosynthesis** (generally temporary devices), and the **prostheses** (definitive devices).

Classification [50]:

- **Inorganic biomaterials:**
  - **Metals**
  - **Nonmetals**:
    Ceramics
    Polymers
    Nanocrystals
    Bone morphogenetic protein (BMP)
- **Organic biomaterials:**
  - Human
  - Animal
  - Plant

1. **Inorganic biomaterials [50]:**
   (a) **Metals and metal alloys:**
   I. **Stainless steels**:
   - Alloys containing iron, the properties vary according to the other components as well as the manufacturing process.
   - Very much used for osteosynthesis and prosthetic devices.
   - Sensitive to corrosion, in particular in the zones of frictions, responsible for ionic release: chronic inflammation with repeated mechanical solicitation.
   - Possible allergies (nickel +++, chromium +).

   II. **Cobalt-chrome-based alloys**:
   - $\approx$ same characteristics as stainless steels, but less wear debris and better friction properties
   - No allergies
   III. **Titanium alloys**:
   - Not very sensitive to corrosion, very good tolerance, low elastic modulus, and thus nearer to bone
   - Poor friction properties
   (b) **Nonmetals:**
   I. **Ceramics [106]:**
   - Material formed by high pressure and temperature (sintering). Compared to traditional ceramics (terra cotta, porcelain, earthenware, glass), new ceramics have specific properties:
     - Corrosion resistance
     - Mechanical, electric and ionic qualities
     - Can be inert or bioactive
   - **Inert ceramics:**
     - **Alumina:**
       Used for alumina-on-alumina combination (THR)
       No oxidation
       No wear debris
       Fragile: microcracks and then fracture (reserved for use on the spherical articular surfaces: head and/or acetabulum)
     - **Zirconia:**
       $\approx$ idem alumina
       Friction coupling possible: zirconia-polyethylene only (zirconia cannot be associated another material of zirconia, alumina, or metal)
       Less and less used: wear of polyethylene, fractures, and osteolysis
   - **Bioactive ceramics [107]:**
     - **Calcium phosphates (hydroxyapatite):**
       Natural mineral component of the bone matrix
       Promotes osteoconduction because it is porous (cf. bone graft page)

© Springer International Publishing AG, part of Springer Nature 2018
G. Chuto et al., *Bone SPECT/CT of Ankle and Foot*, https://doi.org/10.1007/978-3-319-90811-3

Promotes osteoblastosis because it accelerates the recolonization by the bone of the site receiver

Promotes osteointegration because it is gradually reabsorbed and replaced by bone in the receiving site (in 2–3 months for small volumes)

Used in filling material where it is used as support

Used in surface treatment ($\approx$ coating) on a metal substrate (titanium ideally)

II. **Polymers:**
  - Repetition of silica or carbon molecules.
  - **Polyethylene (PE):**
    – Used mainly as a component in friction coupling, liner of acetabular cups in hip arthroplasties.
    – Good resistance.
    – Wear (++), releases small debris that can induce inflammatory reactions: macrophagic activation and osteolysis (granulomatous lesion).
    – One increases the degree of reticulation of polyethylene (length of chain) to increase resistance and to decrease wear.
  - **Polymethacrylic acid (PMMA):**
    – Surgical bone cement, used in particular for the anchoring of hip prostheses, or vertebroplasties and kyphoplasties. Can be used as filling but to avoid because the bone will not take over
    – Allows immediate stability by sealing the prosthetic implant for a quick return to weight bearing
    – Disadvantages: difficulties redoing a cemented implant, extraction of cement
  - **Polylactic and polyglycolic acids:**
    – Used as suture wires, bioabsorbable fixation devices
    – Resorbable, in 6 weeks to 6 months

III. **Nanocrystals [106]:**
  - **Calcium phosphate nanocrystals:**
    – Viscous paste, used in filling for spongy defects (Nanostim®).
    – Nanocrystals provide a large contact surface with the bone, which accelerates osteoinduction and the resorption of the material by macrophages/osteocytes (in 1–2 months).

IV. **Proteins:**
  - **Bone morphogenetic protein (BMP):**
    – Cytokines of the transforming growth factor B family (TGFb)
    – Play a part in the recruiting stem cells from the bone marrow for the osteoblastic line
    – Produced by DNA recombination from hamster ovary cells (rhBMP).

2. **Organic biomaterials [50]:**
  (a) **Human** (cf. bone graft page)**:**
    I. **Autograft**
    II. **Allograft**
  (b) **Animal:**
    I. **Xenograft**
  (c) **Plant:**
    I. **Coral**:
      - Raw [106]:
        – Made of purified calcic crystals.
        – Certain corals have a regular porous structure similar to spongy bone.
        – Certain corals are very dense, similar to cortical bone.
      - Ceramized (treated by sintering)

Bone Grafts

Definitions [107]:
- Osteoconduction: guiding bone tissue growth on the graft site. Nonspecific mechanism, requires that the graft is porous.
- Osteoinduction: capacity of the graft to stimulate undifferentiated cells of the receiving site so that they are differentiate into osteogenic cells.
- Direct osteogenesis: osteoblasts are already present on the graft and immediately participate in osteogenesis. By definition, this capacity exists only for bone autografts, which use fresh tissue.

Bone autograft [50, 107]: reference technique

- Tissue comes from the patient.
- Fresh tissue.

- Contains spongy bone, all the necessary bone-forming growth factors and osteoblasts.
- Types: cortico-spongy graft (iliac crest), spongy graft (from boring), vascularized transplant (fibula).
- Size: <3 cm.
- Bone graft capacities:
  - Osteoconduction: yes
  - Osteoinduction: yes
  - Direct osteogenesis: yes

Bone allograft [50, 107]: for a segmentary loss of substance >6 cm

- Tissue comes from another patient.
- Non-fresh tissue: requires a bone bank, the graft can be:
  - Freeze-dried: simpler to preserve but more friable and hard to shape, is not appropriate for grafts that are too large that are likely to be fractured
  - Fresh-frozen: more logistics involved, more solid and shapable graft to be adapted to the patient
- Safe tissue: physical (irradiation) and chemical treatment to eradicated infectious risks (HIV, hepatitis, etc.) and risk of rejection. Tx is essential but contributes to making the graft more brittle.
- Contains spongy bone.
- Bone graft capacities:
  - Osteoconduction: yes, surface (good on surface, limited inside)

- Osteoinduction: no
- Direct osteogenesis: no

Bone substitutes [50, 107] (cf. biomaterials page): These biomaterials are porous to allow osteoconduction. The pores must have a diameter >100 μm. The more porous the substitute is, the more it facilitates the osteoconduction, but the more it is fragile. It always requires protection by osteosynthesis.

- **Inorganic, nonmetallic, containing calcium phosphate:**
  - Ceramics: of calcium phosphate
    Alone
    With silica and sodium (bioglass)
  - Polymers: calcium phosphate cements
  - Nanocrystals: calcium phosphate
- **Organic:**
  - Plant: coral (gross or ceramized), but is not used any more

Enrichment of the material:

- With osteoinductive growth factors: bone morphogenic proteins (BMP)
- With autologous osteogenic cells: harvested from the patient's hematopoietic marrow or fat tissue
- With calcium phosphate ceramics: coating on a metal substrate (e.g., solid trochanterion mass on the femoral stem of a THR)

Complications of bone allografts [107]:
- Direct osteogenesis impossible: consolidation relies only on the capacities of the bone at the receiving site.
- Receiving site bone:
  - Must be of good quality
  - Need of a well-vascularized bed
  - If not: **pseudarthrosis** (Fig. 1)
- Contact between receiver site and graft:
  - Strict
  - If variation of more than 3 mm on more than 50% of circumference: **pseudarthrosis**
- Mechanical stability:
  - Strict

- Micromobility leads to poor neovascularization: **pseudarthrosis**
- Graft size:
  - The longer or wider the graft, the more fragile it is and the less there is osteoconduction in the center of the graft: the graft must be protected mechanically by a solid osteosynthesis.
  - Under these conditions, when the graft takes well, the transmissions of the forces are transmitted to the graft, in particular in the center of the graft which is the most fragile: **stress fracture.**
  - Osteosynthesis with a screw crossing through the graft weakens it and promotes stress fractures.

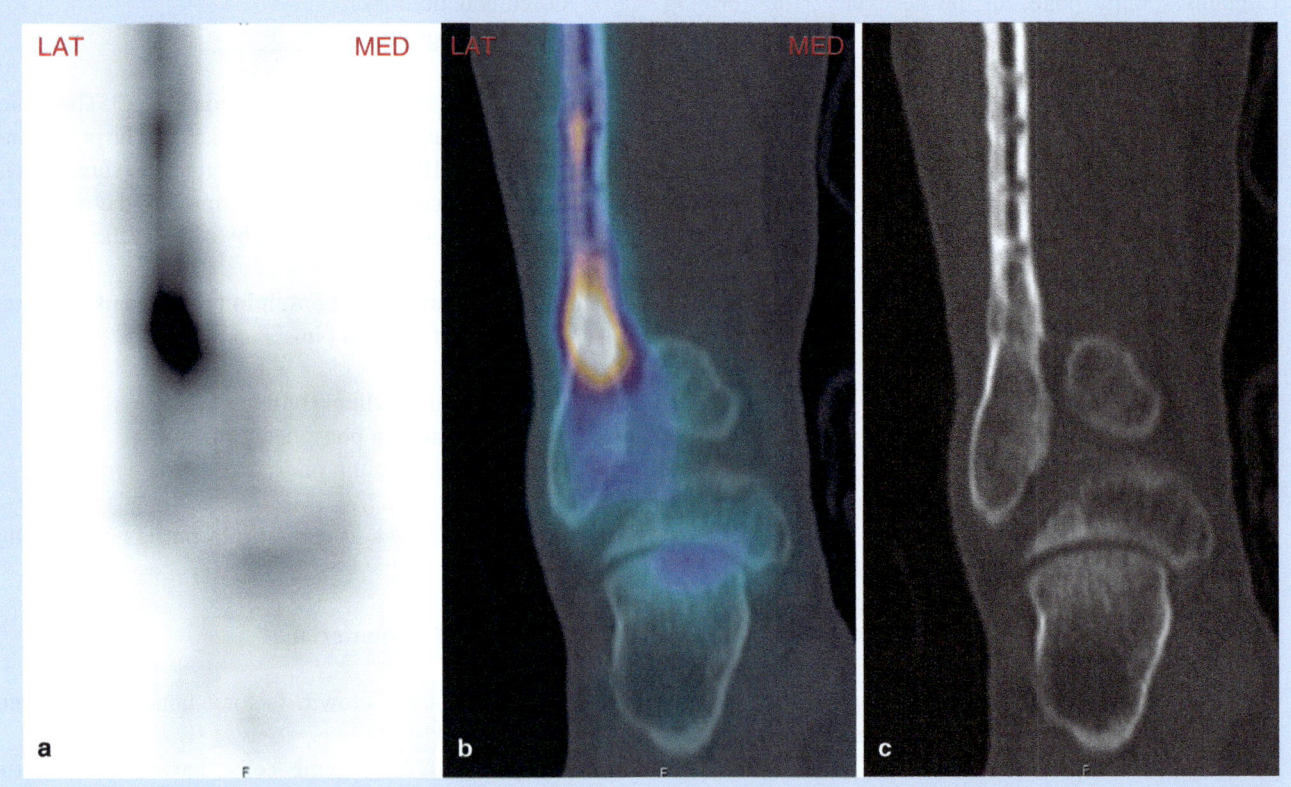

Fig. 1 (**a–c**) Pseudarthrosis on bone graft of the fibula, frontal SPECT (**a**), fused (**b**), and CT (**c**) slices. Osteosynthesis and bone graft on the fibula carried out 16 months prior, ablation of osteosynthesis 4 months prior, persistence of pain: fracture line still visible, with uptake. Note above the marks of the former osteosynthesis with a plate

Osteosynthesis

Classification [50]:

- **Internal osteosyntheses:**
  - Pins
  - Cerclage wires
  - Screws
  - Plates
  - Nails
- **External osteosyntheses:**
  - External fixator

1. **Internal osteosyntheses** (Figs. 2 and 3):
   (a) **Pins**
      - Steel (+++), titanium, or resorbable stems
      - Used for usually temporary or final setting
      - Used for guiding, support for traction
      - Advantages:
        - Low cost
        - Small path
        - Compactness (diameter from 0.8 to 3 mm)
        - Little trauma
      - Disadvantages:
        - Not very stable assembly
        - Does not induce compression
        - Can migrate
   (b) **Cerclage wire**
      - Steel (+++), titanium, or resorbable wires
      - Compression around or through the bone fragment
      - Used for temporary or final setting
   (c) **Screws**
      - Steel (+++), titanium
      - indication:
        - To set bone fragments directly
        - To attach a plate on the bone
      - Advantages: induces compression
      - An isolated screw frequently requires additional stability:
        - Cast
        - Plate (for neutralization)
   (d) **Plates**
      - Steel or titanium
      - Indication: to enable consolidation where there are fracture site constraints

- Possible roles:
  - Neutralization: on bone that is reduced and stabilized by an isolated screw
  - Support: on reduced bone
  - Support and reduction: dynamic compression plate
- Disadvantages:
  - Open reduction: broad pathway, non-respect of the post-fracture hematoma and the periosteal blood supply (all favoring pseudarthrosis)

(e) **Nails (intramedullary nails, or IMN)**
- Steel or titanium
- Hollow (+++) or full tube
- In the medullary cavity of a long bone
- Advantages:
  - Closed reduction (no surgical entry into fracture site)
  - Respect the post-fracture hematoma and the periosteal blood supply, which allows the formation of a good bone callus
- Reamed (+++) or unreamed:

- Benefits of reaming: enlarging of the medullary cavity, more resistant implant, better alignment and larger rate of consolidation
  - Disadvantages of reaming: destruction of the endosteum with ↘ vascularization even if the periosteal blood supply is preserved
- IM nails can be unlocked (to be avoided because of rotation and of telescoping risks) or be locked by proximal and/or distal transmetaphyseal screws)

2. **External osteosyntheses**
   (a) **External fixator:**
   - Temporary or definitive (until bone consolidation)
   - Used for the serious fractures: severe soft tissue damage, wound contamination
   - Cards (or pins for epiphyseal areas):
     - That transpierce the skin, soft tissue, and healthy bone at a distance from the fracture site
     - Connected outside to mechanical apparatuses which allow various assemblies, adapted to each case
   - Advantage: leaves access to soft tissues near the fracture site for local care

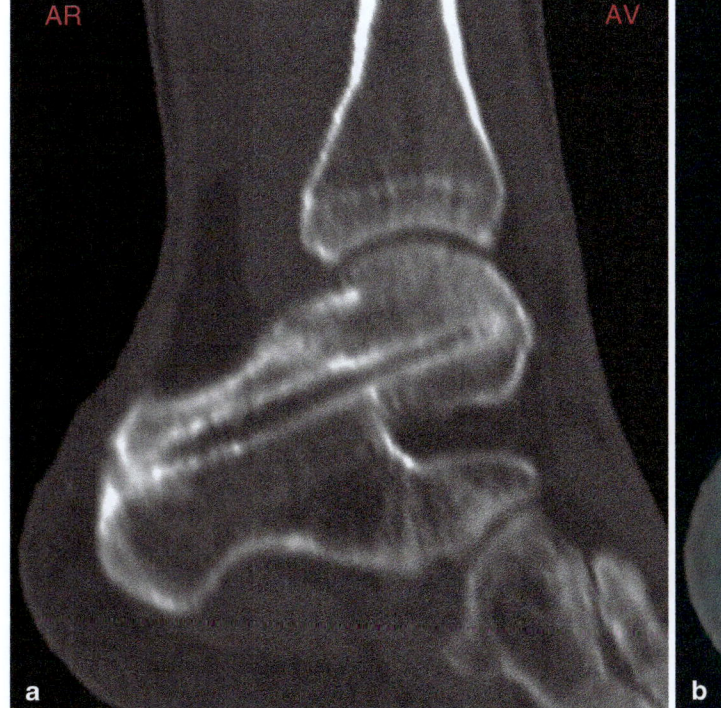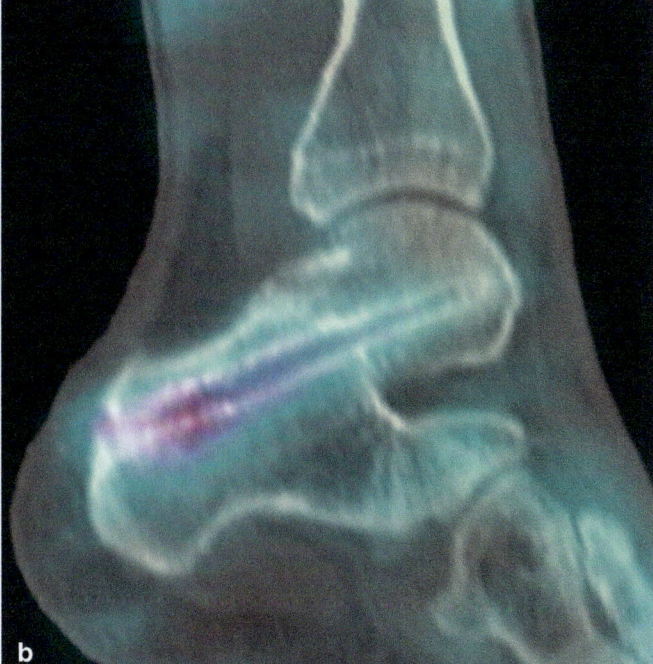

Fig. 2 (**a**, **b**) Subtalar arthrodesis, sagittal CT (**a**) and fused (**b**) slices. Arthrodesis 18 months prior, material removed 6 months prior. Note the subtalar therapeutic ankylosis, without uptake and thus without sign of nonunion. Note that the trace of one of the arthrodesis screws is still visible through the calcaneus and the talus

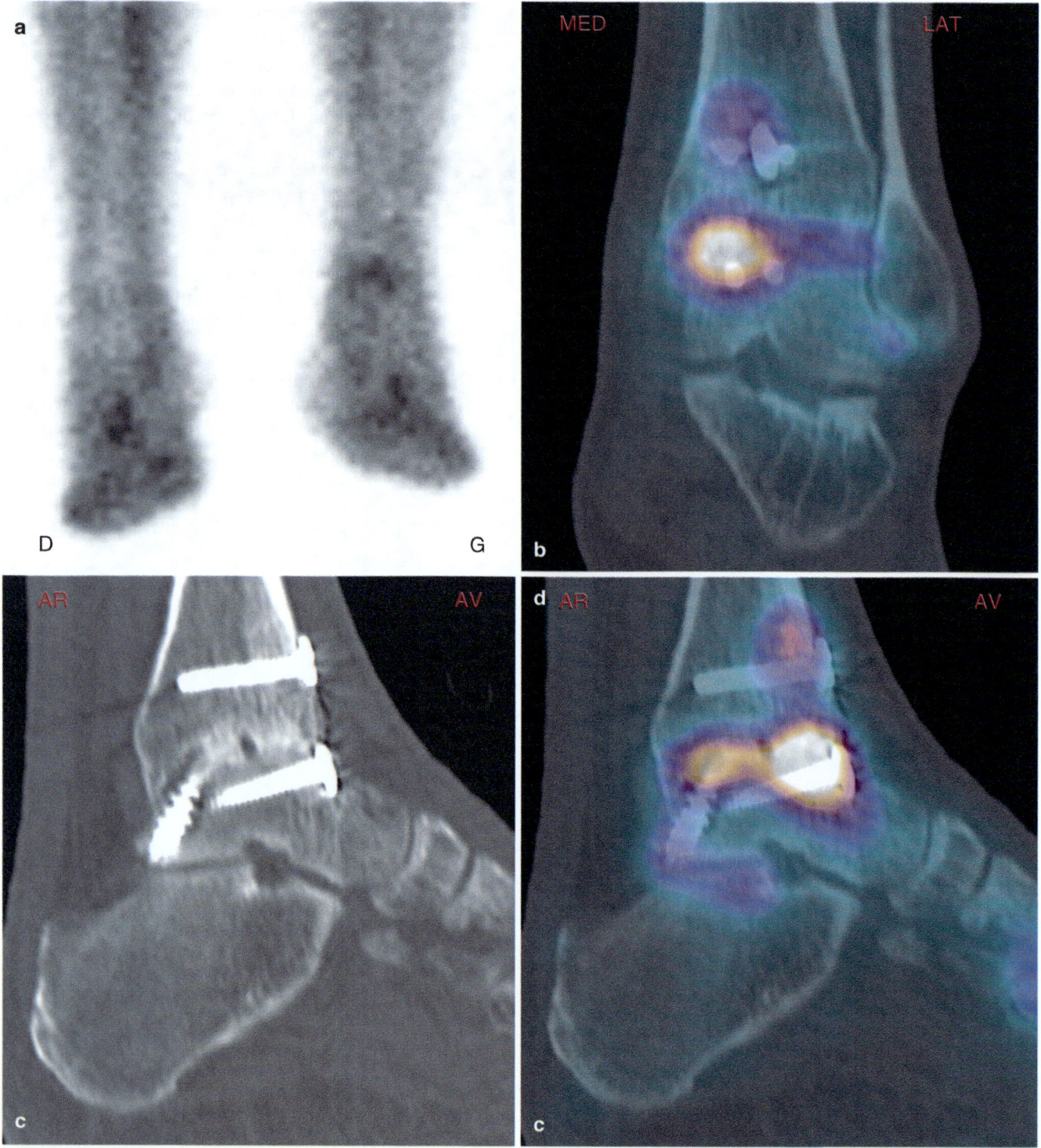

Fig. 3 (**a–d**) Partial nonunion after ankle arthrodesis, front view of blood pool (**a**), fused frontal slice (**b**), sagittal CT (**c**), and fused (**d**) slices. 52-year-old man, left ankle arthrodesis 10 months prior, persistence of pain. Blood pool and delayed activity on the medial part of the ankle in spite of the arthrodesis screws. This aspect is of better prognosis than full uptake on the entire arthrodesis zone. In the follow-up, spontaneous complete fusion

Articular Prostheses

Classification [50]:
- **Cemented/uncemented prosthesis**:
  - Depends on the initial fixation of the prosthesis in the receiving bone site
- **Constrained/unconstrained prosthesis**:
  - Depends on the congruence of the articular interface

1. **Cemented prosthesis**:
   - With stem (for the THA):
     - Out of chromium-cobalt or titanium.
     - Smooth and nonporous: surgical cement is not an adhesive; it fills the interface between the smooth prosthesis and the irregular walls of the medullary canal and distributes pressure in a homogeneous way.
     - Stability: immediate by sealing, a fast resumption of weight-bearing.
     - NB: One cannot speak about primary fixation on a cemented implant, because there is no surface coating and thus no biological secondary fixation.

2. **Uncemented prosthesis**:
   - Treatment of the surface of the prosthesis is necessary, can be:
     - Passive:
       Asperities, porosity, etc.
       Allows osteoconduction
     - Active:
       Osteogenic calcium phosphate ceramics coating
       Allows osteoinduction
   - Primary fixation (mechanical): obtained by peroperational impaction (press-fit). Depends on bone quality: will be excellent in a young subject
   - Secondary fixation (biological integration): good with biological anchoring of the implant

3. **Constrained prosthesis**:
   - Large contact surface for articular interface (e.g., large head and large acetabulum)
   - Good congruence, less instability
   - More constraints on bone anchoring: **loosening**

4. **Unconstrained prosthesis**:
   - Small contact surface for the articular interface
   - Low congruence, more articular play
   - Protects sealing
   - Supports wear of friction couple: **wear debris**

5. **Total ankle arthroplasty (TAA)**:
   - Rare: ≈ 600 TAA/year in France in 2012 [46], compared with the 147,000 THA/year in France in 2010
   - Must preserve maximum bone capital to allow for arthrodesis in the event of failure
   - Requires surfacing of the tibial pilon, of the talar dome +/− the malleoli
   - May be cemented or not
   - Two types:
     - Congruent (constraint)
     - Congruent with a mobile adapter (low constraint)

Complications of prostheses:
- Instability (luxation)
- Loosening, responsible for pain:
  - Loosening is defined by the migration of implant at two radiographic intervals.
  - Border of ≥1 mm is the sign of loosening if it is evolutionary, if not border is considered suspicious and should be assessed on bone SPECT-CT.
  - Impacts the following prostheses:
    Uncemented: border between the bone and the implant
    Cemented: border between the bone and cement and/or spaces between cement and the implant
- Wear:
  - Metal debris: metallosis
  - Polyethylene debris: localized osteolysis (granulomatous lesion) (Fig. 4)
- Fracture
- Heterotopic ossification: +/− responsible for stiffness, pain depending on number and volume
- Infection

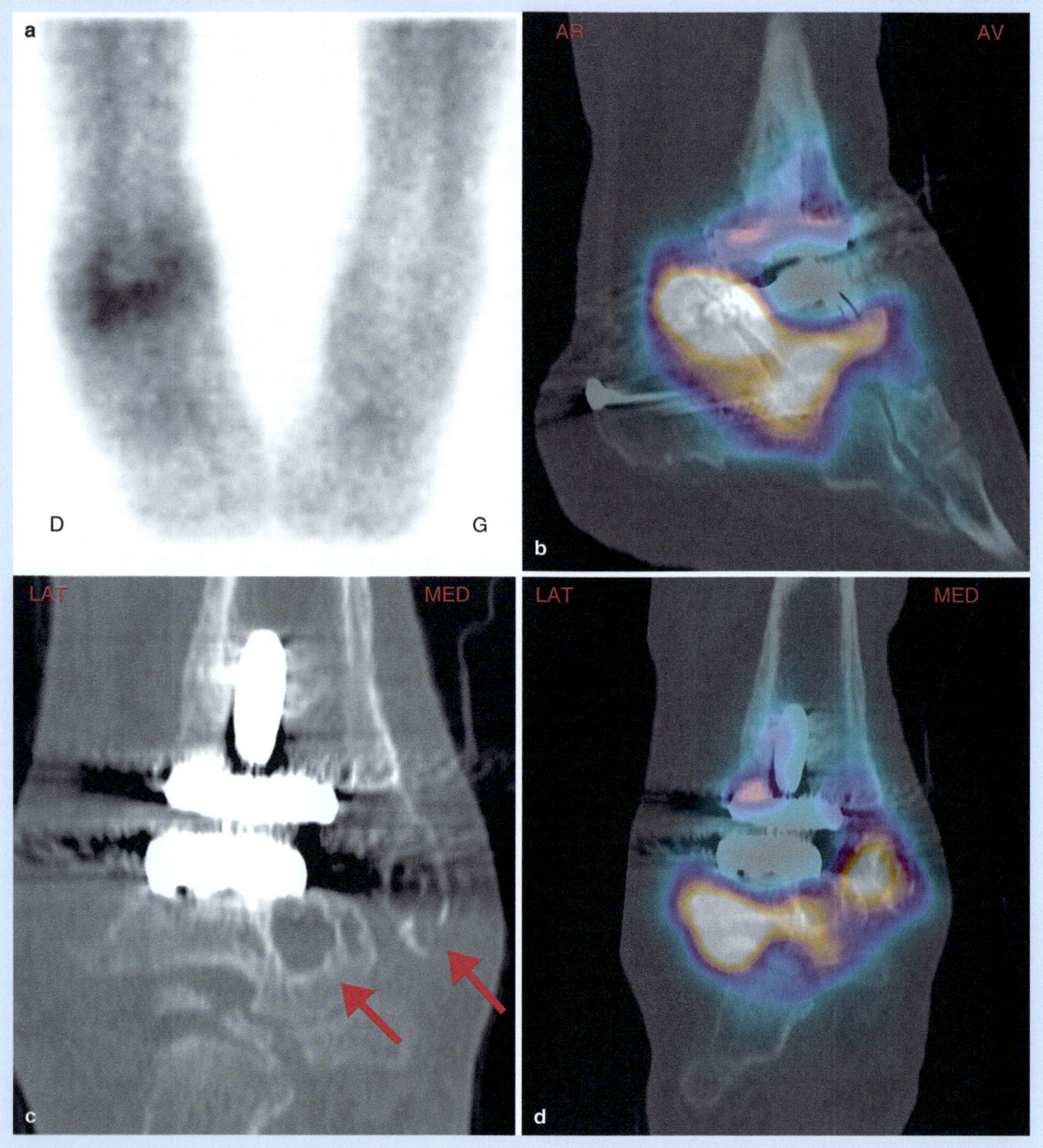

Fig. 4 (**a–d**) Complicated right TAA, front view of blood pool (**a**), fused sagittal slice (**b**), frontal CT (**c**), and fused (**d**) slices. 55-year-old man, right TAA implanted 12 years ago, painful for 1 month. Note the granulomatous lesions on the talus and medial malleolus (arrows), the global uptake of the talus in favor of fracture collapse, and the intense uptake of global subtalar osteoarthritis

Doing a Bone SPECT/CT

We describe the technique used in our service.
Examination is carried out in two or three phases.

Apparatus:
- Hybrid machine combining dual-head gamma camera and a 6-slice CT (Symbia T6, Siemens Healthcare, Erlangen, Germany)
- Low-energy high-resolution collimators
- Energy window: 140 keV +/− 15%

Preparation of the patient:
- None
- Counter-indication: pregnancy

Injection:
- IV
- Disodium hydroxymethane diphosphonate (Technescan) coupled with ^{99m}Technetium (^{99m}Tc-HDP)
- Injected activity: 10 MBq/kg

Phase 1: dynamic (optional)
- Beginning: right before the injection
- Duration: 1 min
- 60 images of 1 s
- Matrix: 64 × 64

Phase 2: blood pool images
- Beginning: 1–2 min post IV
- Duration: 3 min
- Matrix: 128 × 128
- Incidence(s):
  - Front and back: if ankle pain (ankle osteoarthritis, malleolar pain), OLT
  - Plantar: if CRPS I, pain of the forefoot (osteoarthritis of the transverse tarsal or tarsometatarsal joint, sesamoid pathology, stress fracture of the anterior tarsus or toes)
  - External profile: if subtalar pain (osteoarthritis), pain of the calcaneus

Phase 3: delayed images
- Beginning: 2–5 h post IV

Whole body:
- 25 cm/min with reduction of the noise using Pixon® method
- Duration: approximately 7 min

Static images if necessary:
- Duration: 5 min
- Matrix: 256 × 256

SPECT-CT of the foot:
- In decubitus, perfect contention of the feet without any movement, for optimal fusion of the two methods
- Scout:
  - Location
  - Duration: 3 s
- SPECT:
  - Over 360°, in 3° steps, noncircular orbit
  - 32 projections of 15 s on each detection head
  - Duration: 10.5 min
  - Matrix: 128 × 128
  - Zoom: 1
  - Energy window:
    140 keV +/− 15%
    and 126 KeV +/− 15% for estimation of the diffusion
- CT:
  - For attenuation correction and anatomical localization, without injection of ICA
  - Duration: approximately 20 s
  - Tension: 130 kV
  - Optimization of patient dose by CAREDose4D:
    90 mAs reference
    Approximately 10 mAs effective
  - Pitch: 1.25
  - Rotation time: 0.8 s
  - Primary collimation: 6 × 1 mm
  - Field of view: 300 mm
  - Reconstruction of 1.25 mm slices by filtered retroprojection with bone filter (B60) and soft filters (B30)
- Reconstruction of SPECT images:
  - Iterative reconstruction (ordered subset expectation maximum: 3D-OSEM)
    Four iterations
    Eight subsets
    Gaussian post-filter with 5 mm width at half-maximum
  - With attenuation correction, diffusion correction, and depth-dependent resolution compensation

Irradiation:
- *Scintigraphic part:*
  - Effective dose for ^{99m}Tc-HDP:
    4 μSv/MBq [108]
    For a 60 kg patient and an injection of 600 MBq, approximately **2.4 mSv** (compared with the average effective amount of a diagnostic CT of the thorax or abdomen ≈ 5 mSv [109])

- *CT*:
    - Length: 21–28 cm
    - DLP: 45–70 mGy cm
    - IDSV (or $CTDI_{vol}$): 1.4–2.0 mGy
    - Conversion factor specific to each area of the body (K_E) [108]:

      Makes it possible to roughly estimate the effective dose (E) by multiplying it with the DLP: $E = K_E \, DLP$

K_E = 0.0008 mSv/mGy/cm for the extremities (**very weak**, compared with the conversion factor of approximately 0.017 for the thorax, the abdomen, or the pelvis)

Or approximately **0.03–0.05 mSv** by CT examination centered on the feet

References

1. Patel CN, Chowdhury FU, Scarsbrook AF. Hybrid SPECT/CT: the end of "unclear" medicine. Postgrad Med J. 2009;85(1009):606–13.

2. Saha S, Burke C, Desai A, Vijayanathan S, Gnanasegaran G. SPECT-CT: applications in musculoskeletal radiology. Br J Radiol. 2013;86(1031):20120519.

3. Bombardieri E, Frangos S, editors. Nuclear medicine: fusing the ideas of Democritus and Hipocrates: 25 years of the EANM. Vienna: European Association of Nuclear Medicine; 2012.

4. Rodineau J, Besch S. La cheville traumatique: des certitudes en traumatologie du sport. 26e journée de traumatologie du sport de la Pitié-Salpêtrière. Issy-les-Moulineaux: Elsevier Masson; 2008.

5. Bendahou M, Saidi M, Besch S, Khiami F. Traumatisme de la cheville: Springer; 2013.

6. Bergeron Y, Leclaire FL. Pathologie médicale de l'appareil locomoteur. Acton Vale, QC, Canada: Edisem; 2008.

7. Stiell IG, Greenberg GH, McKnight RD, Nair RC, McDowell I, Reardon M, et al. Decision rules for the use of radiography in acute ankle injuries. Refinement and prospective validation. JAMA. 1993;269(9):1127–32.

8. Stiell IG, McKnight RD, Greenberg GH, McDowell I, Nair RC, Wells GA, et al. Implementation of the Ottawa ankle rules. JAMA. 1994;271(11):827–32.

9. Biga N, Rolling A-C. Chirurgie des traumatismes du pied et de la cheville. Lésions récentes et anciennes de l'adulte. Issy-les-Moulineaux: Elsevier, Masson; 2010.

10. Masquelet A-C, Collège français des enseignants en chirurgie de la main, Collège national de chirurgie pédiatrique (France). Orthopédie et traumatologie de l'adulte et de l'enfant: enseignement du deuxième cycle des études médicales. Montpellier: Sauramps Médical; 2008.

11. Vande Berg B, Dosch J-C, Bonnevialle P. Les urgences en pathologie musculo-squelettique—monographie de la SIMS 2012. Montpellier: Sauramps Médical; 2012.

12. Drapé J-L, Guerini H. Imagerie du pied et de la cheville. Issy-les-Moulineaux: Elsevier-Masson; 2010.

13. Liong SY, Whitehouse RW. Lower extremity and pelvic stress fractures in athletes. Br J Radiol. 2012;85(1016):1148–56.

14. Pegrum J, Crisp T, Padhiar N. Diagnosis and management of bone stress injuries of the lower limb in athletes. BMJ. 2012;344:e2511.

15. Lerais J-M. Pathologie articulaire et péri-articulaire des membres: clinique, imagerie diagnostique et thérapeutique. Issy-les-Moulineaux: Elsevier Masson; 2009.

16. Patel DS, Roth M, Kapil N. Stress fractures: diagnosis, treatment, and prevention. Am Fam Physician. 2011;83(1):39–46.

17. Hérisson C, Aboukrat P. Pathologie du medio-pied. Montpellier: Sauramps Médical; 2007.

18. Dobrindt O, Hoffmeyer B, Ruf J, Seidensticker M, Steffen IG, Fischbach F, et al. Estimation of return-to-sports-time for athletes with stress fracture—an approach combining risk level of fracture site with severity based on imaging. BMC Musculoskelet Disord. 2012;13:139.

19. Dobrindt O, Hoffmeyer B, Ruf J, Steffen IG, Zarva A, Richter WS, et al. Blinded-read of bone scintigraphy: the impact on diagnosis and healing time for stress injuries with emphasis on the foot. Clin Nucl Med. 2011;36(3):186–91.

20. Beck BR, Bergman AG, Miner M, Arendt EA, Klevansky AB, Matheson GO, et al. Tibial stress injury: relationship of radiographic, nuclear medicine bone scanning, MR imaging, and CT Severity grades to clinical severity and time to healing. Radiology. 2012;263(3):811–8.

21. Leemrijse T, Valtin B. Pathologie du pied et de la cheville. Issy-les-Moulineaux: Elsevier Masson; 2009.

22. Zengerink M, Struijs PAA, Tol JL, van Dijk CN. Treatment of osteochondral lesions of the talus: a systematic review. Knee Surg Sports Traumatol Arthrosc. 2010;18(2):238–46.

23. Badekas T, Takvorian M, Souras N. Treatment principles for osteochondral lesions in foot and ankle. Int Orthop. 2013;37(9):1697–706.

24. Leumann A, Valderrabano V, Plaass C, Rasch H, Studler U, Hintermann B, et al. A novel imaging method for osteochondral lesions of the talus—comparison of SPECT-CT with MRI. Am J Sports Med. 2011;39(5):1095–101.

25. Ha S, Hong SH, Paeng JC, Lee DY, Cheon GJ, Arya A, et al. Comparison of SPECT/CT and MRI in diagnosing symptomatic lesions in ankle and foot pain patients: diagnostic performance and relation to lesion type. PLoS One. 2015;10(2):e0117583.

26. Wiewiorski M, Pagenstert G, Rasch H, Jacob AL, Valderrabano V. Pain in osteochondral lesions. Foot Ankle Spec. 2011;4(2):92–9.

27. Meftah M, Katchis SD, Scharf SC, Mintz DN, Klein DA, Weiner LS. SPECT/CT in the management of osteochondral lesions of the talus. Foot Ankle Int. 2011;32(3):233–8.

28. Strobel K, Steurer-Dober I, Da Silva AJ, Huellner MW, del Sol Pérez Lago M, Bodmer E, et al. Feasibility and preliminary results of SPECT/CT arthrography of the wrist in comparison with MR arthrography in patients with suspected ulnocarpal impaction. Eur J Nucl Med Mol Imaging. 2014;41(3):548–55.

29. Huellner MW, Strobel K. Clinical applications of SPECT/CT in imaging the extremities. Eur J Nucl Med Mol Imaging. 2014;41(Suppl 1):S50–8.

30. Vaseenon T, Amendola A. Update on anterior ankle impingement. Curr Rev Musculoskelet Med. 2012;5(2):145–50.

31. Chicklore S, Chicklore S, Gnanasegaran G, Vijayanathan S, Fogelman I. Potential role of multislice SPECT/CT in impingement syndrome and soft-tissue pathology of the ankle and foot. Nucl Med Commun. 2013;34(2):130–9.

32. Ribbans WJ, Ribbans HA, Cruickshank JA, Wood EV. The management of posterior ankle impingement syndrome in sport: a review. Foot Ankle Surg. 2015;21(1):1–10.

33. Russo A, Zappia M, Reginelli A, Carfora M, D'Agosto GF, La Porta M, et al. Ankle impingement: a review of multimodality imaging approach. Musculoskelet Surg. 2013;97(Suppl 2):S161–8.

34. Peyrou P, Moulies D. Les "fausses entorses" de l'adolescent. J Traumatol Sport. 2006;23(2):96–104.

35. Laredo J-D, Wybier M, Bellaïche L. Savoir faire en radiologie ostéo-articulaire n° 8 (2006). Montpellier: Sauramps Médical; 2006.

36. Singh VK, Javed S, Parthipun A, Sott AH. The diagnostic value of single photon-emission computed tomography bone scans combined with CT (SPECT-CT) in diseases of the foot and ankle. Foot Ankle Surg. 2013;19(2):80–3.

37. Prieur A-M. Maladies systémiques et articulaires en rhumatologie pédiatrique. Paris: Flammarion Médecine-Sciences; 2009.

38. Carlioz H, Seringe R. Orthopédie du nouveau-né à l'adolescent. Issy-les-Moulineaux: Masson; 2005.

39. Diméglio A, Hérisson C, Simon L. Le Pied de l'enfant et de l'adolescent. Paris: Masson; 1998.

40. Finidori G, Glorion C, Langlais J. La pathologie épiphysaire de l'enfant. Groupe d'étude en orthopédie pédiatrique, éditeur. Montpellier: Sauramps Médical; 2003.

41. Bouysset M, Delmi M, Morvan G. Le pied et cheville de la clinique aux examens complémentaires. Montpellier: Sauramps Médical; 2014.

42. Morvan G, et al. Le pied—monographie de la SIMS 2011. Sauramps Médical: Montpellier; 2011.

43. Scharf SC. Bone SPECT/CT in skeletal trauma. Semin Nucl Med. 2015;45(1):47–57.

44. Coughlin MJ, Baumfeld DS, Nery C. Second MTP joint instability: grading of the deformity and description of surgical repair of capsular insufficiency. Phys Sportsmed. 2011;39(3):132–41.

45. Monographie AFCP n°5—SOFCOT 2009. Montpellier: Sauramps Médical; 2009.

46. Monographie AFCP n°9—SOFCOT 2013. Montpellier: Sauramps Médical; 2013.

47. Bard H, et al. Le tendon et son environnement—monographie de la SIMS 2013. Montpellier: Sauramps Médical; 2013.

48. Laredo J-D, Wybier M, Bousson V, Parlier C, Petrover D, Miquel A. Savoir faire en radiologie ostéo-articulaire n° 15 (2013). Montpellier: Sauramps Médical; 2013.

49. Dorland. Dictionnaire médical bilingue français-anglais, anglais-français—28ème édition. Issy-les-Moulineaux: Elsevier-Masson; 2008.

50. Masquelet A-C. Chirurgie orthopédique. Principes et généralités: Masson; 2012.

51. Kamina P. Anatomie clinique—membres—tome I. 4ème. Vol. tome I. Paris: Maloine; 2009.

52. Matin P. The appearance of bone scans following fractures, including immediate and long-term studies. J Nucl Med. 1979;20(12):1227–31.

53. Jolles-Haeberli B. Manuel pratique de chirurgie orthopédique. Issy-les-Moulineaux: Elsevier Masson; 2013.

54. Riise ØR, Kirkhus E, Handeland KS, Flatø B, Reiseter T, Cvancarova M, et al. Childhood osteomyelitis-incidence and differentiation from other acute onset musculoskeletal features in a population-based study. BMC Pediatr. 2008;8:45.

55. Ceroni D, Belaieff W, Cherkaoui A, Lascombes P, Schrenzel J, de Coulon G, et al. Primary epiphyseal or apophyseal subacute osteomyelitis in the pediatric population: a report of fourteen cases and a systematic review of the literature. J Bone Joint Surg Am. 2014;96(18):1570–5.

56. Haidar R, Der Boghossian A, Atiyeh B. Duration of post-surgical antibiotics in chronic osteomyelitis: empiric or evidence-based? Int J Infect Dis. 2010;14(9):e752–8.

57. Zimmerli W, Trampuz A, Ochsner PE. Prosthetic-joint infections. N Engl J Med. 2004;351(16):1645–54.

58. Lentino JR. Prosthetic joint infections: bane of orthopedists, challenge for infectious disease specialists. Clin Infect Dis. 2003;36(9):1157–61.

59. Lew DP, Waldvogel FA. Osteomyelitis. Lancet. 2004;364(9431):369–79.

60. Lhotellier L. Infections précoces d'origine opératoire, résultats et indications des nettoyages associés à une antibiothérapie. Rev Chir Orthop. 2002;(88):166–8.

61. Cotten A. Imagerie musculosquelettique. Pathologies générales. Issy-les-Moulineaux: Elsevier Masson; 2013.

62. Gelber AC. In the clinic. Osteoarthritis. Ann Intern Med. 2014;161(1):ITC1-16.

63. Kellgren JH, Lawrence JS. Radiological assessment of osteoarthrosis. Ann Rheum Dis. 1957;16(4):494–502.

64. Clegg DO, Reda DJ, Harris CL, Klein MA, O'Dell JR, Hooper MM, et al. Glucosamine, chondroitin sulfate, and the two in combination for painful knee osteoarthritis. N Engl J Med. 2006;354(8):795–808.

65. Pagenstert GI, Barg A, Leumann AG, Rasch H, Müller-Brand J, Hintermann B, et al. SPECT-CT imaging in degenerative joint disease of the foot and ankle. J Bone Joint Surg Br. 2009;91(9):1191–6.

66. Knupp M, Pagenstert GI, Barg A, Bolliger L, Easley ME, Hintermann B. SPECT-CT compared with conventional imaging modalities for the assessment of the varus and valgus malaligned hindfoot. J Orthop Res. 2009;27(11):1461–6.

67. Barg A, Pagenstert GI, Horisberger M, Paul J, Gloyer M, Henninger HB, et al. Supramalleolar osteotomies for degenerative joint disease of the ankle joint: indication, technique and results. Int Orthop. 2013;37(9):1683–95.

68. Claassen L, Uden T, Ettinger M, Daniilidis K, Stukenborg-Colsman C, Plaass C. Influence on therapeutic decision making of SPECT-CT for different regions of the foot and ankle. Biomed Res Int. 2014;2014:927576.

69. Kretzschmar M, Wiewiorski M, Rasch H, Jacob AL, Bilecen D, Walter MA, et al. 99mTc-DPD-SPECT/CT predicts the outcome of imaging-guided diagnostic anaesthetic injections: a prospective cohort study. Eur J Radiol. 2011;80(3):e410–5.

70. Kim H-R, So Y, Moon S-G, Lee I-S, Lee S-H. Clinical value of (99m)Tc-methylene diphosphonate (MDP) bone single photon emission computed tomography (SPECT) in patients with knee osteoarthritis. Osteoarthr Cartil. 2008;16(2):212–8.

71. Dieppe P, Cushnaghan J, Young P, Kirwan J. Prediction of the progression of joint space narrowing in osteoarthritis of the knee by bone scintigraphy. Ann Rheum Dis. 1993;52(8):557–63.

72. Scott DL, Wolfe F, Huizinga TWJ. Rheumatoid arthritis. Lancet. 2010;376(9746):1094–108.

73. Aletaha D, Neogi T, Silman AJ, Funovits J, Felson DT, Bingham CO, et al. 2010 rheumatoid arthritis classification criteria: an American College of Rheumatology/European League Against Rheumatism collaborative initiative. Ann Rheum Dis. 2010;69(9):1580–8.

74. Kim JY, Cho S-K, Han M, Choi YY, Bae S-C, Sung Y-K. The role of bone scintigraphy in the diagnosis of rheumatoid arthritis according to the 2010 ACR/EULAR classification criteria. J Korean Med Sci. 2014;29(2):204–9.

75. Orphanet: Arthrite psoriasique [Internet]. [cité 2 juill 2015]. http://www.orpha.net/consor/cgi-bin/OC_Exp.php?Lng=FR&Expert=40050.0

76. Gladman DD, Chandran V. Observational cohort studies: lessons learnt from the University of Toronto Psoriatic Arthritis Program. Rheumatology (Oxford). 2011;50(1):25–31.

77. Taylor W, Gladman D, Helliwell P, Marchesoni A, Mease P, Mielants H, et al. Classification criteria for psoriatic arthritis: development of new criteria from a large international study. Arthritis Rheum. 2006;54(8):2665–73.

78. Scarpa R, Cuocolo A, Peluso R, Atteno M, Gisonni P, Iervolino S, et al. Early psoriatic arthritis: the clinical spectrum. J Rheumatol. 2008;35(1):137–41.

79. Tan AL, Tanner SF, Waller ML, Hensor EMA, Burns A, Jeavons AP, et al. High-resolution [18F]fluoride positron emission tomography of the distal interphalangeal joint in psoriatic arthritis—a bone-enthesis-nail complex. Rheumatology (Oxford). 2013;52(5):898–904.

80. Raza N, Hameed A, Ali MK. Detection of subclinical joint involvement in psoriasis with bone scintigraphy and its response to oral methotrexate. Clin Exp Dermatol. 2008;33(1): 70–3.

81. Tan AL, McGonagle D. Psoriatic arthritis: correlation between imaging and pathology. Joint Bone Spine. 2010;77(3):206–11.

82. Gastaldi G, Ruiz J, Borens O. [Charcot osteoarthropathy: don't miss it!]. Rev Médicale Suisse. 2013;9(389):1212, 1214–20.

83. Recommandations pour la pratique clinique. Prise en charge du pied diabétique infecté. SPILF, Texte court [Internet]. [cité 1 juill 2015]. http://www.infectiologie.com/site/medias/_documents/consensus/pieddiabetique2006-court.pdf

84. Khodaee M, Lombardo D, Montgomery LC, Lyon C, Montoya C. Clinical inquiry: what's the best test for underlying osteomyelitis in patients with diabetic foot ulcers? J Fam Pract. 2015;64(5):309–10, 321.

85. Palestro CJ. 18F-FDG and diabetic foot infections: the verdict is... J Nucl Med. 2011;52(7):1009–11.

86. Teh J, Berendt T, Lipsky BA. Rational Imaging. Investigating suspected bone infection in the diabetic foot. BMJ. 2009;339: b4690.

87. Malhotra R, Chan CS-Y, Nather A. Osteomyelitis in the diabetic foot. Diabet Foot Ankle. 2014;5.

88. Treglia G, Sadeghi R, Annunziata S, Zakavi SR, Caldarella C, Muoio B, et al. Diagnostic performance of fluorine-18-fluorodeoxyglucose positron emission tomography for the diagnosis of osteomyelitis related to diabetic foot: a systematic review and a meta-analysis. Foot (Edinb). 2013;23(4):140–8.

89. COFER. Rhumatologie. France: Elsevier; 2011.

90. Goebel A. Complex regional pain syndrome in adults. Rheumatology (Oxford). 2011;50(10):1739–50.

91. Borchers AT, Gershwin ME. Complex regional pain syndrome: a comprehensive and critical review. Autoimmun Rev. 2014;13(3):242–65.

92. Chronic Foot Pain—American College of Radiology Appropriateness Criteria 2013 [Internet]. [cité 19 août 2015]. https://acsearch.acr.org/docs/69424/Narrative/

93. Algodystrophie ou syndrome douloureux régional complexe de type I [Internet]. [cité 15 juin 2015]. http://mn-net.pagesperso-orange.fr/doc/docos/rhumato/vasculaire/algodystrophie.html

94. Harden RN, Bruehl S, Stanton-Hicks M, Wilson PR. Proposed new diagnostic criteria for complex regional pain syndrome. Pain Med. 2007;8(4):326–31.

95. Harden RN, Bruehl S, Perez RSGM, Birklein F, Marinus J, Maihofner C, et al. Validation of proposed diagnostic criteria (the "Budapest Criteria") for Complex Regional Pain Syndrome. Pain. 2010;150(2):268–74.

96. Varenna M, Adami S, Rossini M, Gatti D, Idolazzi L, Zucchi F, et al. Treatment of complex regional pain syndrome type I with neridronate: a randomized, double-blind, placebo-controlled study. Rheumatology (Oxford). 2013;52(3):534–42.

97. Moon JY, Park SY, Kim YC, Lee SC, Nahm FS, Kim JH, et al. Analysis of patterns of three-phase bone scintigraphy for patients with complex regional pain syndrome diagnosed using the proposed research criteria (the "Budapest Criteria"). Br J Anaesth. 2012;108(4):655–61.

98. Roddy E, Mallen CD, Doherty M. Gout. BMJ. 2013;347:f5648.

99. Dalbeth N, Fransen J, Jansen TL, Neogi T, Schumacher HR, Taylor WJ. New classification criteria for gout: a framework for progress. Rheumatology (Oxford). 2013;52(10):1748–53.

100. Feneis DW. Lexique illustré d'anatomie. Paris: Médecine-Sciences Flammarion; 2007.

101. Alberts BM, Johnson A, Lewis J, Le Sueur-Almosni F, Berthaut I, Kamoun P. Biologie moléculaire de la cellule. Paris: Flammarion Médecine-Sciences; 2004.

102. Vander AJ, Widmaier EP, Raff H, Strang KT. Physiologie humaine: les mécanismes du fonctionnement de l'organisme. 6ème. Montréal; Paris: Chenelière éducation: Maloine; 2013.

103. Rouvière H, Delmas A, Delmas V. Anatomie humaine: descriptive, topographique et fonctionnelle. Tome III. 15ème. Paris: Masson; 2002.

104. Os surnuméraires et sésamoïdes du pied. SIMS—GEL Contact n°17 [Internet]. [cité 28 août 2015]. http://www.sims-asso.org/uploads/pdfs/gelcontact/9/1.pdf

105. Brasseur J, Morvan G. Echographie de la cheville et du pied. Montpellier (Hérault): Sauramps Médical; 2012.

106. Mainard D. Les substituts de l'os, du cartilage et du ménisque en 2011. SOFROT—SOFCOT. Paris: Romillat. p. 2011.

107. Monographie AFCP n°8—SOFCOT 2012. Montpellier: Sauramps Médical; 2012.

108. Brix G, Nekolla EA, Borowski M, Noßke D. Radiation risk and protection of patients in clinical SPECT/CT. Eur J Nucl Med Mol Imaging. 2014;41(Suppl 1):S125–36.

109. Biswas D, Bible JE, Bohan M, Simpson AK, Whang PG, Grauer JN. Radiation exposure from musculoskeletal computerized tomographic scans. J Bone Joint Surg Am. 2009;91(8):1882–9.

Index

The manufacturer's authorised representative in the EU is Springer
Nature Customer Service Centre GmbH, Europaplatz 3, 69115 Heidelberg,
Germany. If you have any concerns regarding our products, please
contact ProductSafety@springernature.com

Printed and bound by CPI Group (UK) Ltd, Croydon, CR0 4YY
27/04/2026
02097672-0002